Social Work and Child Abuse

D0139790

While social work practice with child abuse is a well-documented topic, this revised edition of *Social Work and Child Abuse* actually challenges and changes the focus of existing literature. Instead of concerning itself with the ways in which the task of preventing and detecting child abuse can be more effectively undertaken, it presents a critical analysis of the task itself.

There has been much new guidance and regulation since the first edition of *Social Work and Child Abuse* was published in 1996, making this a timely new edition. With a brand new introduction and conclusion, this fully revised text discusses:

- the implications of the Victoria Climbié Inquiry, the Laming Report, the Green Paper Every Child Matters and the 2004 Children Act
- the 1989 Children Act and the conflicting duties of the social worker to prevent and intervene in child abuse and also to promote 'the family'
- the emergence of official discourses of prevention, treatment and punishment
- the 1975 Children Act and the role of moral panic.

Concluding with a call for the full implementation of the UN Convention on the Rights of the Child to strengthen the child-protection system by giving children and young people a much stronger voice, this book is essential reading for all professionals in social and probation work, and for students in social work, social policy and criminology.

Dave Merrick has extensive experience in Child Protection, as a child protection social worker, as a Children's Guardian and as a Principal Inspector for Children's Services. He is currently serving a secondment as the National Children's Rights and Participation Development Officer for the Children and Family Court Advisory and Support Service (CAFCASS). He also lectures on social policy for the Open University.

Social Work and Child Abuse

Still walking the tightrope?

Second edition

Dave Merrick

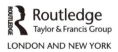

Routledge
Taylor & Francis Group

LONDON AND NEW YORK

First published 1996
by Routledge

This edition published 2006
by Routledge
2 Park Square, Milton Park, Abingdon, Oxon OX14 4RN

Simultaneously published in the USA and Canada
by Routledge
270 Madison Ave, New York, NY 10016

*Routledge is an imprint of the Taylor & Francis Group,
an informa business*

© 1996, 2006 Dave Merrick

Typeset in Times New Roman by
Newgen Imaging Systems (P) Ltd, Chennai, India
Printed and bound in Great Britain by
The Cromwell Press, Trowbridge, Wiltshire

British Library Cataloguing in Publication Data
A catalogue record for this book is available
from the British Library

Library of Congress Cataloging in Publication Data
A catalog record for this book has been requested

ISBN10: 0-415-35414-5 (hbk)
ISBN10: 0-415-35415-3 (pbk)
ISBN10: 0-203-00086-2 (ebk)

ISBN13: 978-0-415-35414-1 (hbk)
ISBN13: 978-0-415-35415-8 (pbk)
ISBN13: 978-0-203-00086-1 (ebk)

Contents

Acknowledgements

This book would not have been possible without the assistance, both direct and indirect, of many people. The children, young people and their families and carers with whom I have worked in social work over a 30-year period have taught me so much, as have my colleagues in social work. Students and staff at the University of the West of England, the Open University and the University of Birmingham have also taught me a great deal. In addition, my colleagues in the Children and Family Court Advisory and Support Service (CAFCASS) have been a great source of learning and encouragement.

Professor Gill Hague has provided a great deal of support, including reading and commenting upon draft chapters. My children, Keiran and Cassie, have provided me with love, support and perspective throughout this period. Needless to say, any mistakes, confusions, gaps or silences are all my own.

Introduction to 2006 edition

It was with no small degree of trepidation that I decided to reconsider the argument that I presented in the first edition of this book, originally published in 1996. Apart from anything else, there is a temptation to 'let sleeping dogs lie', because, if a reader can tolerate another hackneyed cliché, 'matters had moved on'. However, after serious consideration I genuinely felt that this was not an option that was open to me. I will endeavour to outline my reasons for this conclusion immediately below.

Whilst the arguments of the book have been in the public domain for 10 years, and whilst it has sold, and still sells well, within an academic community, and is cited in other works on the subject, either as recommended reading (e.g. Corby 2006) or in terms significant work on the subject (e.g. Goldson, Lavallette and McKechnie 2000; Hill and Tisdall 1998), I nevertheless feel that the essentials of the argument have not been fully grasped by policy makers in the field. Clearly this would only matter if there were important points that are missed as a consequence of this. After due consideration, I feel that this is the case. In order to illustrate the reason for this it is necessary to briefly outline the central argument of the book.

A KEY QUESTION

When I conducted fieldwork amongst child and family social workers for the original book, one single observation seemed to me then and now to pose a very key question, and it was this: 'if a person on probation goes out and commits an armed robbery, or shoots or rapes someone, nobody says, "What was the probation officer doing?"' The point is that when things go tragically wrong on a social worker's caseload, especially if a child is involved, then it seems as if *everybody* wants to know what the *social worker* was doing. Why is this? How did this arise? Perhaps more importantly, will it continue to arise?

This book contends that the answer lies in the conflicting duties placed upon social workers in over 70 years of childcare legislation. The point is simply that however unfair media coverage of such events may sometimes seem the sad fact is that there is a real question to be asked about what went wrong. The book argues that it is the simultaneous duty to prevent, and detect, child abuse and also to rehabilitate children with parents/caretakers or 'the' family, which will at times produce situations where social workers are focused to a greater extent on any one of these statutory duties at the expense of the others. This leaves them vulnerable to the periodic charge that they are either intervening to too great or too little an extent – as in, for instance, the case of Maria Colwell, and many other subsequent cases, on the one hand, and the Cleveland cases and many other subsequent cases on the other.

The book suggests that it is the tension between a legislative duty to intervene into 'the family' where there is believed to be a risk of 'significant harm' to the child, and also the duty to promote 'the family' as the best place to look after children, which necessarily involves the prediction and prevention of child abuse and the provision of support to families, which leads periodically, episodically, but nevertheless inevitably to the kind of opposite outcomes involved in the Colwell and Cleveland cases.

In other words, it is not too little or too much intervention which is alone the major issue; it is rather the imperative legislative duty of social workers to intervene for often very differing and conflicting reasons which leads inevitably at times to, quite simply, the wrong intervention at the wrong time, and this can contribute to tragic outcomes for children. However, so interwoven are these conflicting demands that it is often only with the benefit of hindsight that this becomes clear.

Since the first edition of the book was written there have been subsequent childcare tragedies, such as, on the one hand, that of Victoria Climbié, which is a horrifying example of insufficient intervention, and, on the other hand, a number of high-profile cases of successful appeals against convictions for the abuse, even murder, of children. These appeals have often been based on what was at the time considered to be expert evidence from expert witnesses, for example, paediatricians. For instance, Sally Clark, Angela Cannings and Donna Anthony have all had convictions overturned. Such contradictory situations are perhaps indications that prima facie, at least, the argument of the book is worth restating and reconsidering.

Hence this new edition will offer a new chapter which considers the case of Victoria Climbié, and the subsequent public inquiry, chaired by Lord Laming, the Green Paper, entitled 'Every Child Matters', and the Children Act 2004, which represents the Government's legislative response to the

Laming Report (2003). The chapter suggests that policy makers have not taken the argument on board, and that, if the inherent tensions within the legislation were more fully recognised this could potentially considerably improve child-protection services. Whilst policy makers and decision makers routinely make the observation that social workers are in a difficult position in which they are 'damned if they do and damned if they don't', they are never able to articulate the historical and discursive roots of this dilemma. In addition the chapter argues that, in not acting upon Lord Laming's recommendation concerning the implementation of the UN Convention on the Rights of the Child, the government missed an opportunity to potentially protect children and young people by raising their status and standing in society as a whole and by strengthening the duty of all professionals involved to engage with them directly and to actively seek and consider their opinions in relation to any matter that impacts upon them.

Since 10 years has elapsed since the first edition of this book it seems appropriate to update a reader upon my own subsequent professional biography. Over that past 10 years, whilst I have continued to teach for the Open University, I have, in the main, been more focused on social-work practice and policy. I have worked as the Principal Inspector for Children's Services for the City of Bristol and as a Children's Guardian (previously Guardian Ad Item). My current role is as the National Children's Rights Development Worker for the Child and Family Court Advisory and Support Service (CAFCASS) in England.

These roles (perhaps particularly that of Children's Guardian, the task of which is to make recommendations to a Family Court in relation to the wishes and feelings of the child or young person concerned, their best interests and whether making any particular statutory order is better than making none at all) are important in the field of child protection. Hence I feel that I bring to this reconsideration a very current practice and policy-based perspective, as well as a more detached 'academic overview'. I hope that this will make a contribution to at least clarifying some of the complex dilemmas involved in child protection and potentially improving child-protection policy and services as a result of that. The following chapter outline will assist the reader in understanding the structure of the book.

OUTLINE OF CHAPTERS

Chapter 1: Teaching or preaching?

This chapter considers the extent to which literature which claims to base itself on an understanding of the history and practice of contemporary social work addresses the dilemmas raised by social workers in practice. The work reviewed was written from a socialist, or a Marxist, or an explicitly feminist and/or anti-racist perspective. While the chapter recognises the importance of these texts in posing important questions in relation to the history and current practices of social work and their welcome recasting of traditional social-work approaches, it nevertheless argues that there is a tendency in many of them to assert and assume rather than to argue. In addition there is a tendency at times to be formulaic and reductionist.

The chapter also argues that in relation to statutory social work, and working with children and families in that context, which necessarily involves a focus upon childcare legislation and policy, these texts tend to be particularly weak. Few of them devote sufficient attention to these issues, and those of them that do so do not consider in detail or in depth the historical emergence of the particular and increasingly central issue of child abuse. It is this absence which produces responses which are overly formulaic or reductionist in their analysis. I suggest that all of this frequently lacks an appropriate degree of empirical detail. This fact leads me to turn to a more detailed consideration of potential methods through which more of such detail might be provided.

Chapter 2: Questions of theory

Chapter 2 outlines the theoretical position on which the book's arguments are based. It first briefly considers Rojek, Peacock and Collins (1988), who endeavour to construct an approach to social work based upon discourse analysis. The chapter suggests that the authors overstate the degree of vulgarity of both Marxism and the feminisms, which their work is in part a response to and in part a reaction against. It is also suggested that the type of social work which they advocate, and term *subjectless social work*, as well as their view of discourse analysis upon which it is premised, also have a strong tendency to reductionism. This points to the necessity of attempting to develop a less reductionist account of the work of both Marx and Foucault. Emerging from that theoretical encounter are the specific ways in which this book attempts to apply elements and versions of discourse analysis and elements of contemporary theories of ideology in understanding the discourse contained in the various documents which are considered in Chapters 3–6.

Chapter 3: Still walking the tightrope?

This chapter considers the tragic case of Victoria Climbié and the public inquiry that followed. Lord Laming chaired the inquiry and the report was published in January of 2003. The government responded by producing the Green Paper *Every Child Matters*, and this formed the basis of the Children Act 2004. The Green Paper and the new Act will also be considered, both in the context of the original argument of the book and of course in its own terms. It concludes that because Lord Laming sees the 1989 Children Act and the social-work contradictions in which it is embedded as sound and as not in need of analysis, this leaves the competing discourses, and the resultant conflicting duties of social workers, intact if not entirely unexamined. It focuses instead on the issue of the better implementation of the 1989 Children Act. This reinforces the relevance of the following chapter which considers that Act. The chapter also argues that the Government, in declining to act on the implementation of the UN Convention on the Rights of the Child, missed an opportunity to strengthen the voice and the rights of children and young people within the child-protection system.

Chapter 4: The 1989 Children Act – a significant shift?

The 1989 Children Act is the focus of Chapter 4. This Act was represented as a major overhaul of family and childcare law. Hence the chapter considers the extent to which the boundaries of intervention between the law and 'the family' were redrawn by the Act. It concludes that the central role of social workers in terms of statutory responsibility for the prevention, rehabilitation and detection of child abuse remained largely untouched, and in some important senses social workers and their agencies were further centralised in the issue. This calls forth a necessity to consider the ways in which, historically, particular discourses and ideologies have contributed to the production of the dilemmas that contemporary social work faces.

Chapter 5: A stitch in time – the men from the ministry

This chapter considers the work of the Children's Branch of the Home Office in the 1920s and 1930s and the emergence in official circles of a discourse of prevention. Hence this chapter attempts, through the scrutiny of the Home Office Reports on the work of the Children's Branch of 1923, 1925 and 1939 and also the Report of the Departmental Committee on Sexual Offences Against Children and Young Persons 1925, and the 1927 Departmental Committee on the Treatment of Young Offenders, to uncover the emergence of this discourse. It then considers the Curtis Committee (1946), both the Final Report and the Interim

Report, which called for training in childcare and suggested its form, content and duration.

Chapter 6: The 1960s and the short-lived 'triumph' of treatment

This chapter considers the legislation of this later period against the analysis in the Chapter 5 by outlining the position that the radical social-work texts take in relation to the Ingleby Report (1960), the Children and Young Persons Act of 1963, and the White Papers *The Child, the Family and the Young Offender* of 1965 and *Children in Trouble* (1968). The chapter then analyses the discourse in all of these documents and considers it in relation to the view that this period represented the triumph of the discourse of treatment over that of punishment. It argues that, while this period represents the *high-water mark* of the discourse of treatment, it is nevertheless not accurate to see this as the *triumph* of treatment. This is important because it illustrates that even in this period there remained considerable ambiguity in the statutory duties of social workers between prevention and treatment on the one hand and detection and punishment on the other.

Chapter 7: Moral panic and Maria Colwell

This chapter critically examines the question of the role played by moral panic in rendering child (physical) abuse as a matter for urgent attention, and also in the production of the 1975 Children Act. It should be emphasised at the outset that the chapter does not deny the existence of such a panic. What is at stake is a question of emphasis between, on the one hand, a view which sees this Act as representing a radical break from previous practice and, on the other hand, a view which sees a significant degree of continuity, in part produced by the retaining within this legislation of ideologies and discourses which played a key part in the construction of previous legislation. A careful analysis of this dichotomy, which attempts to give each side its proper weight, provides a fuller and more accurate picture of the emergence of both the current concerns in relation to child abuse and their discursive and legislative roots.

Chapter 8: Back to the future

The concluding chapter summarises and restates the argument of the book and provides a potential answer to the 'key question' which motivated the initial research. Furthermore, it considers the implications of all of this for contemporary social-work practice.

Chapter 1

Teaching or preaching?

This chapter reviews the social-work literature which claims to base itself on a critical understanding of the political history of contemporary practice in social work. The work reviewed was written from a socialist, or a Marxist, or an explicitly feminist and anti-racist perspective. These are important because, apart from standard social-history texts, they are the only texts which claim to offer any historical analysis of social work. In addition they are important because they were, and are still in many quarters, influential in social work, particularly in social-work education.

A major problem to be confronted in reviewing this literature is concerned with what should be included. Included are texts which have the words 'radical social work' in their title. Also included are texts which do not, but which nevertheless are addressed to social workers in the context of a political/historical analysis of their activity; therefore books are included which focus on specific issues and attempt to develop and outline a social-work practice in that context, for example, anti-racist social work, feminist social work, women and social work. The earlier work is reviewed first, except where a later text takes up an issue which I consider to have been neglected by an earlier text.

RADICAL SOCIAL WORK

Bailey and Brake's (1975) *Radical Social Work* a collection of essays ranging from an introductory essay by the editors attempting to analyse the historical development of social work in the welfare state, to an article relating to the endeavour to develop a radical social-work practice.

The debt to classical Marxism

The editors' introduction, while appearing to some extent to distance itself, is in its essentials classically Marxist. It suggests that

> Welfare can be allowed to develop with the cooperation of the working class movements, because it does not challenge ideologically the fundamental nature of capitalist democracy. This is not to argue that these benefits should be rejected as reformist, nor that the benefits gained in class struggle through the thrust of trade union power should be belittled but . . . as long as the unions act and others act as pressure groups within the state context, they tend to sustain rather than undermine the established situation.
>
> (Bailey and Brake 1975: 2)

Even though these authors are concerned not to belittle particular gains made by the working class in struggle, an orthodox Marxism is at the root of this work nevertheless. This orthodoxy has been subsequently criticised for its gaps and silences and its apparent assumptions of a unified and singular working class, always having the same material interests, however unconscious of them that they (or even it) may at times be. Of course, as further work in this field emerged there were attempts to criticise and respond to these gaps and silences, and these endeavours will also be considered in this chapter.

This text was an attempt to move towards improvement on the often very apolitical and oppressive social-work practices of the day. To do so it was necessary to convince its audience that there was at least the possibility of such a practice. To do this it was necessary first to deal with the cruder versions of social-control theory. The following illustrates the way in which this was attempted:

> To see social workers, in short, as simply the willing henchmen of the ruling class in its exercise of social control is to take an undialectical view. It overestimates the rationality and monolithic nature of the capitalist state in its ability to determine in detail the activities of an occupation.
>
> (Leonard 1975: 49)

The attraction, and point, of such an argument is that it creates a space within which social work can be seen as at least potentially positive. There is the potential at least for a progressive practice. But this then begs the question of the nature of the practice itself; it is here, particularly in this early work, that radical social work is weak. Social work is, in essence, an active and not an analytical profession. Something always has to be done, and therefore theory, if it is to be taken seriously, must be readily applicable in practice.

It is not strictly true to suggest that there is no practice on offer, even in this early text, but it is true to say that it is limited. In the first place any radical social-work practice faces a dilemma that its more conventional competitors do not. Quite simply, at its base there is a desire to develop a social-work practice that itself seeks to be a part of, and even facilitate, a transcending of the macro-social conditions which it believes make a major, if not the major, contribution to the distress that the consumers of social-work services face. At the same time it is concerned to meet the real and immediate needs of those who come to a social-work office in the hope of receiving help for what is often a specific, and to those people, an essentially personal problem. The kernel, therefore, of any practice that makes a claim to be radical, or in later texts socialist, anti-racist, etc., must be its ability to address and utility in addressing *both* of these seemingly opposite poles.

Two of the articles in Bailey and Brake (1975) explicitly attempt to grapple with this dilemma. Leonard (1975) offers one such attempt. In his conclusion he is disarmingly candid; he admits that 'it will be clear that radical social work is a long way from being able to formulate a coherent paradigm of theory and practice' (Leonard 1975: 61).

An orientation to a radical social-work practice

Leonard offers what he considers to be an *orientation* to radical practice. In doing so, he offers four *aims* of radical social work. The first is 'education', that is, essentially consciousness raising of one's service users.

He advises the *linking of people to 'systems'*, for example, one should be conscious of the potential isolation of service users and attempt to empower them by, where possible and appropriate, assisting them to link with pressure groups and self-help groups.

He also advises the *building of counter systems*, either within or outside the existing system. This may involve trade-union work, pressure-group activity, counter-information systems, informal support groups, etc., for social workers and service users or both in combination, and he suggests that radical social workers should work both *in* and *against* the welfare structures of the capitalist state (see pp. 55–9).

Leonard also advises *group conscientisation*, which involves working with clients and others in an 'action system' to achieve change (p. 60). In addition he urges radical social workers to develop organisational, planning and administrative skills since, quite apart from anything else, none of the aforementioned aims could be achieved without them.

The project and the practice of radical social work

In responding critically to the above it is important to separate the questions of the ultimate project (which appears to be to facilitate, if not a revolution, then certainly a process of criticism and contestation, which is thought of as contributing to such an outcome) from the question of a specific method of social work.

In relation to the former, what is clear is that the analysis is explicitly Marxist, although it is not possible to state the precise philosophical basis of the Marxism involved because it is not fully visible. An inspection of the index of the book reveals that there are two references to Lenin, ten to Marx and Engels, and none to Stalin or to Stalinism or theoretical attempts to overcome it. In fairness, Leonard, for instance, points out that, 'many radical social workers...have little taste for theory, and are deeply suspicious of the mystifying and divisive effects of theorizing' (p. 47). Nevertheless, he insists that if radical activity within social work is to avoid becoming 'mere unreflective activism', then it must take seriously Lenin's proposition that, 'without a revolutionary theory there can be no revolutionary movement' (Lenin 1963 *What is to be Done?* quoted by Leonard 1975: 47).

In relation to the social-work practice he advocates, it could be argued that his advice could equally well be taken by any social-work practice, and indeed it could be argued that it is currently mainstream, and in some aspects was mainstream at the time. It was often possible therefore for social workers to respond by suggesting that radical social-work practice, in so far as it was elaborated at all, and when stripped of revolutionary rhetoric, simply seemed to amount to good social-work practice.

Marxism, radical social work and the critique of social democracy

Bolger *et al.* (1981), *Towards Socialist Welfare Work*, is more elaborate in its attempt to develop a radical social-work practice, and is also more explicit about the form of Marxism upon which it is predicated. The book, as its title implies, is an endeavour to encourage 'socialist experiments in welfare practice' (see Leonard in the editor's introduction, p. xiii).

The book offers a critique of social democracy and social democratic approaches to welfare. It sees social democracy as an 'impressively strong ideology'. It is strong because it is, on the one hand, 'structured into the fabric of institutions through social policy' and, on the other hand, it is 'an ideology used to study these institutions' (p. 9). It is, however, in the view of these authors flawed because

> The crucial factor here is the social democratic conception of politics. The Labour Party in Great Britain has failed to construct a democratic relationship between the state welfare apparatus and the working class. Welfare reforms are imposed from 'above'. They are then run by professionals... We can detect a social democratic fear of the working class – a fear that they are not actually capable of being involved in the administration of state services. In fact this probably reflects a more fundamental fear that the working class is racist, sexist, and individualist and does not actually want the state services that are being imposed on it!
>
> (p. 12)

This is thought to be of help in understanding the electoral defeat of the Labour Party in 1979. On this analysis the defeat represented a rejection by a large portion of the working class of these services, which had been imposed in the way outlined earlier, and which, therefore, had no democratic base. The question of the democratic relationship between the welfare state and the working class is the key to the book. Essentially the book is a call to (radical) social workers to attempt to both provide elements of, and to prefigure the missing democratic element. Since this analysis underpins the work, it is not difficult to infer the essential message to practitioners which, when stripped of all rhetoric, involves their attempting wherever possible to facilitate and construct this missing democratic alliance.

A critical analysis of the above would involve a number of issues, for example, the seemingly homogeneous nature of the working class, and the role of class struggle pure and simple in the production and reproduction of particular political outcomes. Even if this is taken as given, there would still be the crucial question of the differential experiences of oppression within the working class, for example, the specific oppression of racism, of gender, etc. There is also a related issue concerning the make-up of the populations who are the subjects/objects of intervention by the welfare state, since there is a distinction to be made between the working class as a whole and those of them who at any given time constitute the overwhelming bulk of the 'client' population.

When considering these authors' analysis of British childcare legislation, it is clear that they take a particular view of social democracy and its relationship to the working class, for instance of the 1969 Children and Young Person's Act. They suggest that, 'thus the . . . Act was forced onto the statute book by a Labour government whose respect for "expertise" capable of "serving the nation as a whole" had led it to a dependency on Fabian academics and social work professionals' (p. 90). The passage continues to complain that the Labour Party did not develop a 'broadly based political alliance'.

The position outlined earlier in relation to the activities of the Labour Party, Fabian expertness and the presence/absence of the working class in the construction of British child care legislation is criticised in later chapters of this book. Much work in this field offers, in essence, aversion of, or is a development of, the earlier analysis. (See, in addition to Bolger et al. (1981), Parton (1985), Pitts (1988), Frost and Stein (1989), all of which are critically evaluated in subsequent chapters of this book.)

There are two texts which give more attention to the fact that the working class is far from homogeneous. They are London Edinburgh Weekend Return Group (1980) and Jones (1983). These texts are too early to take in the debate in relation to the changing nature of the working class: for example, episodic part-time employment, the question of whether there is in existence an underclass of unemployed or underemployed people who are permanently accorded only a 'client' status and in which women and black people are more commonly placed than are white men etc. Nevertheless, these texts do offer a different emphasis from that of the texts so far reviewed. Since Jones (1983) is explicitly engaged with the text reviewed earlier, it is appropriate to take his work before that of the London Edinburgh Weekend Return Group (1980).

STATE SOCIAL WORK AND THE WORKING CLASS

Jones (1983) does not endeavour to provide a radical social-work practice. Rather his work is focused on the attempt to come to an understanding of the historical development of state welfare. It is again an essentially Marxist analysis and it is explicitly said in the editor's introduction to be pursuing the same project as the texts reviewed earlier. The book illustrates the way in which the state has been in large measure successful in fragmenting the poor from the rest of the working class. However, social workers, via their experience of the deprivation of their clients and their own altruism/liberalism, are constantly at risk of 'contamination' and therefore become unreliable and difficult employees. The book is concerned with the way a 'class fraction' (p. xiii), that is, state employees, have been used to manage the working-class poor. Jones therefore considers the question of how social-work training and social-work management endeavours to control and police its own recruits.

Jones differs from the texts reviewed earlier in a number of respects, for instance their characterisation of the welfare apparatus as essentially social democratic. He points to

> The repressive social security, racist nationality laws, the appalling increase in poverty and despair, the manner in which community care policies are reinforcing the subordination of women and the dependants for whom they care to new depths of misery, the accelerating drift to more punitive policies with respect to young offenders, are just some of the issues currently facing social workers and demanding attention.
>
> (p. 7)

The book is richer in historical detail and empirical research than the texts reviewed earlier. Chapters 2 and 3 consider the clients of social work and the way in which the state has attempted to deal with the problems which they pose. Chapter 4 considers the relationship of social-work clients to the whole of the working class. The second half of the book (Chapters 5–8) considers social workers themselves and

> Seeks to demonstrate the many difficulties and problems which have confronted the state in employing concerned and often liberal social workers and directing them to intervene deeply into the lives and circumstances of some of the most deprived and impoverished victims of contemporary society.
>
> (p. 8)

Democracy is also central in this text, as in the texts previously reviewed, because this demand arises from the growing recognition that many of the welfare services created under social democracy concentrated power in the hands of unaccountable 'professional experts' – which was a key reason why so many of the working-class consumers of such services found them to be patronising and stigmatising (p. 155).

However, Jones, in common with Simpkin (1983), remembers that 'there are within working class culture long standing antagonistic strands to the client population', and he points out that, in the absence of a 'vibrant mass socialist movement', democratisation may not be in the interests of clients, since it may be that power would shift only from 'unaccountable experts' to 'representatives of the moral majority' (Jones 1983: 155).

The development of social-work professionalism

Jones is at his most interesting and innovative in the chapters which concern the historical development of the social-work profession and the question of social-work training. Both in his published and unpublished work he charts, via empirical historical research, what he sees as the development of the beginnings of social-work professionalism.

In doing so he focuses upon the activities and the discourses of the Charity Organizing Society (COS). It is worth outlining some of this in detail, since it also helps to illustrate the way in which early social work played a part in stigmatising its 'client' population via the construction of the categories of deserving/undeserving. This fact must play a part in the continued animosity towards 'claimants' that Jones, following Simpkin (1983), recognises.

The discourse of the COS was ideologically situated in the context of class struggle and in its conflicts with the Fabian Society and other positions to the left of itself. The COS, in claiming to have developed a 'scientific' understanding of pauperism, produced the key claim that pauperism could therefore be prevented. What this involved was selectivity and individualisation. In adopting this position they were well in the mainstream of pro-capitalist political thought.

Jones sees the COS, via its claim of a scientific approach to poverty, as being involved in a 'struggle for closure' which involves both establishing their own particular view of social work as the dominant view and in recruiting, training and also controlling their own recruits. On this analysis the idea of professionalism becomes essentially an occupational strategy and he quotes Weber in support of this.

> When we hear from all sides the demand for the introduction of regular curricula and special examinations, the reason behind it is not a suddenly awakened 'thirst for education' but the desire for restricting the supply of these positions and their monopolization by owners of educational certificates.
>
> (Weber 1948, quoted in Jones 1983: 84)

He also quotes a director of the COS School of Sociology who suggests that

> The terms in which our truths are expressed often belong to a passed age; have we not all been at times uneasily conscious that the mere appeal to fundamental principles has lost much of its force, and that these principles must be recast,... clothed in a new language, for it is unquestionably true that the new generation is receptive enough, but as always demands a new preparation of its food.
>
> (Urwick 1904, quoted in Jones 1983: 91)

What is on offer above is not a re-examination of 'fundamental principles' but a re-launch of them 'clothed in a new language': Jones illustrates a continuity in this strategy of using different language in order to relaunch already existing but differently named ideas. Forty-three years later the assertion is made that

> [Social science and research] make it respectable to talk about 'factors in social pathology' instead of the undeserving poor; 'community stimulation' instead of getting lonely people along to the Settlement social; 'providing positive incentives to socially acceptable behaviour' instead of helping with the Brownie pack; 'psychopathic personalities' instead of hopeless scroungers; 'rehabilitating the socially maladjusted' instead of trying to reform anyone or anything. The essential rose remains unchanged by this change in names, but if anyone is helped thereby to see more clearly, to think more deeply, to diagnose more truly, and to treat more effectively, then this change, and all others that succeed it are all to the good.
>
> (Younghusband 1947, quoted in Jones 1983: 91)

Essentially, what Chris Jones offers is an account of the development of professionalism within social work, in which he sees continuity from the early days of the COS to the present. This is a continuity within which social-work education socialises carefully selected recruits into the social-work profession and in which social-work managements continually have to police their employees to avoid contamination. One of the advantages of the book is that it presents detailed historical evidence of this process.

A critical analysis of the text would, however, raise the following points. There is a risk, in reading Jones, that one may reduce the whole of social work to social-work professionalism, but not all of social-work activity can be simply equated with its own occupational strategy. It is important to remember that within every line of development there was competition and contestation between differing forms of philanthropy, between differing forms of 'collectivism' – for example, Fabianism, early feminism – and between differing forms of resistance. There is little in Jones that illustrates the complexity of the number of overlapping traditions that went into the formation of social work: for example,

- *Philanthropy*, which may take the form of agitation for or against legislation or particular practices, as well as taking the form of simple charity in the context of a gift. Philanthropy cannot of itself be described as a strategy because it was not in itself homogeneous.
- *Direct social activism*, for example, Robert Owen, Mary Carpenter; often grouped very loosely around the Social Science Association in the 1850s and 1860s, for example, the settlement movements.
- *Reformers within social administration*, that is, reformers who were a part of the poor law administration, for example, Edwin Chadwick.
- *Fabian agitation and permeation*, social work was ultimately absorbed into the very state machinery the COS feared. While the COS may have produced the role of the professional 'expert' and laid the ground for social work professionalism, the Fabians, at first indirectly and later very directly, made an important contribution to this process.

There is also the question of professionalism itself. Chris Jones illustrates the cynicism in much of the manoeuvring of the COS and also of later social-work educators. However, the work is vulnerable to an emphasis which sees the social-work profession as emerging in the main from the activities of social workers and social-work educators themselves. It is sometimes as if they chose their task, chose their language, chose their strategy and were, apart from their problematic recruits, largely successful. This begs a number of important questions. In the first place, if one considers the 'traits' approach to professionalism, it becomes clear that social work fails to meet a number of the criteria for acceptance as a profession. Quite clearly, for instance, social work does not control its own decision making, since it remains in very large measure a state-defined activity. It cannot be said either that the knowledge base of social work can be considered as being on a par with that of doctors or lawyers. Indeed, much of its knowledge base is borrowed from other disciplines and professions. Hence social work cannot be considered as a fully developed profession on the basis of a traits analysis of professions.

The idea of a continuum between occupations, semi-professions and professions is of use in understanding the position of social work. For instance, there is a clear tension between social workers' position within an organisation and a desire for professional status. It is a tension between administrative imperatives and professional autonomy. Of course this does not mean that occupations and semi-professions do not aspire to professional status. However, against this must be set the question of 'proletarianisation'. Aspiring to professional status is one thing, achieving it is quite another.

Crucially, social work is mediated by the state. It is not the case that either the social worker or even his or her supervisors and managers define consumer need any more than it is the consumers who define their own needs, or even which of them should be met. The state has been the crucial mediator in not only controlling but also defining a social worker's role. This is particularly clear in relation to the development of British childcare legislation, with which this book is concerned. The contradictory and often near impossible role which has been assigned to social workers via childcare legislation is documented in the pages of this book.

Also the level of professional judgement and autonomy permitted to social workers is limited. There is supervision, and management, though it is also true that managements may make use of professional values to induce self-regulation (see Larson 1977).

In each of the texts reviewed there is, at both an implicit and explicit level, the critique of professionalism outlined earlier, though Jones is the more explicit and empirical. This raises an important point about the function within these texts of a critique of professionalism. There is an important sense in which this critique is politically motivated.

If professionalism can be seen as purely an occupational strategy, which is flawed, then the call to social workers to become active in their trade unions, which is presented as both a more effective, and a less elitist, occupational strategy, will have more resonance. This, in addition will bring them into closer contact with the labour movement, which is part of the radical strategy that these texts offer. Bolger *et al.* (1981) have in mind the official trade-union movement, perhaps reflecting some commitment on their behalf to the strategy of the British Communist Party, whereas with Jones (1983) it is the rank-and-file trade-union movement, which perhaps reflects his distance from the same.

This leads to an overemphasis on professionalism within social work as always and everywhere, potentially, if not in reality, both cynical and successful. It needs to be remembered that there are many times when it is neither. This is not to say that what Chris Jones documents is not true; it is merely to remember that there is also some altruism involved in the concept of professionalism and that the profession itself, for the reasons outlined earlier, is not simply the brainchild of its own membership. His view of the matter also overlooks the fact that there is evidence to suggest that even where social work plays a potentially very controlling role, for example, in cases of child cruelty or child abuse, appeals are sometimes made to social workers for an intervention. For instance, Gordon (1989), working from the actual case records of a child-cruelty agency in Boston, USA at the turn of the century, documents cases where women appealed to social workers to intervene in order to protect their children from the violence of men. This does not square with a view of professionalism that is always self-seeking and cynical, though of course this is not to say that there are not times when it is that. The absence of a more nuanced consideration of these issues leaves his text vulnerable to crude and potentially unhelpful reading.

IN AND AGAINST THE STATE

The London Edinburgh Weekend Return Group (1980) was first published as a pamphlet. It was then subtitled 'Discussion Notes for Socialists'. It differs from the texts reviewed earlier in two important respects. In the first place, while it is also explicitly socialist, it nevertheless attempts to move beyond the organised left which 'provides no answers' (p. 134). Some of the group are 'women and feminists' and they say that 'for us the struggle – to change relations within society is not just against capitalism but against sexism as well' (p. 4).

Prefigurative practice and the need for a better theory of the state

The London Edinburgh Weekend Return Group (1980) is of the view that the state is important, but that a new and better theory of it is required. The kernel of this new theory is the recognition of two differing 'senses' of the state. This involves the recognition of the state both as a form or process of social relations and as an institution (see pp. 58–9). The focus for day-to-day struggle is against the state in the former sense or, more precisely, against the form or process of social relations which it perpetuates. By this means the question of gender and race becomes central to socialist politics.

However, the authors do not have a strategy to offer and what they offer instead is a need to develop a tentative feeling for principles. The book concludes by offering four such principles:

1 Socialist politics must be rooted in people's own experience.
2 Socialism cannot be built without a vision of what is possible.
3 Our whole lives are subject to capitalism.
4 Socialism is about transforming power relations, not about capturing power.

(pp. 143–5)

The authors, in their final paragraph, counterpose 'practical experience in struggle' against 'utopian dreaming' and again urge the necessity to 'forge our own form of organisation'. This is because 'a struggle in our own way is the only possible point of departure for a world we can live in on our own terms. The future must be ours and not theirs, and we must make it now' (p. 147).

What the authors attempt is essentially a forerunner of endeavours to contribute to the process of the construction of (though the term is not used) a 'rainbow coalition' out of autonomous social movements engaged together 'in struggle' and in the process developing new and better forms of organisation based on a politics rooted in the lived experience of the participants.

The notion of prefigurative practice derives from the work of Antonio Gramsci. However, it is perhaps important to note that the Gramscian borrowing is selective. Gramsci may well have been an innovative Marxist, but a Marxist he remained. Throughout his life he was a committed Communist Party member. Hence in Gramsci there was a theory for the transition from capitalism to socialism, and this centrally involved the Communist Party. Gramsci himself suggests that

It has already been said that the protagonist of the new Prince could not in the modern epoch be an individual hero, but only the political party. That is to say, at different times, and in the internal relations of various nations, that determining party which has the aim of founding a new type of state (and which was rationally and historically created for that end).

(Gramsci 1978: 147)

This is important because the traditions that these authors criticise have a theory of transition, of which they are critical. The prescription these authors advance has none. It is perfectly reasonable to abandon all political parties, and all existing theories of the transition from capitalism to socialism, if they are found wanting. Nevertheless it seems to me that to borrow Gramsci, but to divorce the political party from his theories, leaves a serious gap. It is as if 'the struggle' (albeit in new forms) is in itself enough.

Socialism and the question of power

This links with the authors' fourth principle, that is, 'Socialism is about transforming power relations not about capturing power' (London Edinburgh Weekend Return Group 1980: 143–5). This separation is perhaps a little glib. Surely there will be times, or even a time, when in order to transform a power relationship, the power itself may need to be captured. The fact that not everybody will obey orders is a transformation in a power relationship, but in the real and brutal world of political violence, the question of who gives the orders is at least as important and is, of course, a question concerning the possession of power.

This does not mean that alternative and better forms of organisation should not be sought, but it is to note that such endeavours cannot stand in themselves as the route to socialism. This is quite apart from the question of what might constitute socialism in the wake of the revolutionary defeat of Stalinism, and social democracy appearing to have abandoned what little commitment to socialism it had.

On the other hand the resistance, for instance, to the war in Iraq, a resistance which was often shunned by the official labour movement, and which was carried out in the streets, by organised protests, and which included significant sections of the population who were not 'organised' in the myopic and traditional socialist sense of that word, is testimony, were such testimony needed, to the fact that new forms of struggle and contestation can and do develop, and that they can be vibrant and successful.

THE TASKS OF SOCIALISTS AND THE TASKS OF SOCIAL WORK

An important question in relation to the texts reviewed earlier is the fact that there appear to be times when the 'macro' socialist project overtakes and subordinates the 'micro' individual project of simply helping people, which is at base what state services, that is, social work etc., ought to be about and, in however a contradictory way, are often in fact about. People are often at their very lowest ebb by the time they turn to a social worker, and in such situations notions of democratic alliances, fighting back, collective strength etc., seem, and often are, quite simply, albeit sadly, beside the point.

This is particularly clear in a statutory context. It is no simple matter to take a child into care. To do that democratically is perhaps, in the end, impossible. One of the fault lines of all of the literature so far reviewed is that the prescriptions for practice offer something which might well be possible in the 'easier' cases, but not in the more intractable and difficult ones. Unfortunately it is often precisely these more difficult situations that social workers confront.

A further important point is that in the texts reviewed earlier there is reticence about dealing with individuals as individuals. The suspicion of 'case work' and 'individualism' gives rise to the risk of a reading in which the attempt to understand individuals as individuals is seen as in some sense unprogressive.

A gap in Marxism – a materialist theory of personality?

Leonard (1984) recognises this reticence and attempts to fill what he sees as a 'gap in Marxism'. What is lacking is 'detailed attention to the dialectic between the individual and the social order, whereby the former is socially constructed, but within a context of struggle and resistance' (p. 5).

The analysis is more theoretically sophisticated than those presented above, leaning as it does upon Freud, Lacan, Althusser etc. It acknowledges a debt to socialist feminism, and recognises the fact of racism. However, for all its attempts at detail, it runs the risk of all grand theory. In the end it lacks specificity. For all the recognition of unique biography, and for all its endeavour to avoid a crude determinism, there remains a homogeneity in the context of class, gender and race. This is illustrated when it is suggested that

> If we are to help ourselves and others to work for an alternative society, then we must try to grasp more fully what we have been required to repress in ourselves in order to become gendered class subjects properly prepared for labour.
>
> (p. 217)

It may be of help to know the ways in which people can be prepared as gendered class subjects, but it does beg the question of whether we are all equally that.

Class–subject positions and collective subjectivities

Gilroy (1987) suggests that 'if it is to continue to be useful, class analysis like class struggle cannot be confined to individuals who occupy positions in the immediate process of production' (p. 32). There is a central reason for this, and it concerns the fact of a large amount of structural unemployment. He asks

> If as Gorz has argued, class membership is increasingly being lived out as 'contingent and meaningless fact', the ground upon which the whole productivist Marxian edifice has been erected is in jeopardy. Where is the radical collective action to come from in the miserable years of crisis and crisis management which await Britain?
>
> (p. 246)

He replies that 'it is likely to arise from those groups who find their collective existence threatened', and he concludes that

> Race must be retained as an analytical category . . . because it refers investigation to the power that collective identities acquire by means of their roots in tradition. These identities, in the forms of white racism and black resistance, are the most volatile political forces in Britain today.
>
> (p. 246)

It is important, as Gilroy's book demonstrates, to avoid a myopic, ethnocentric and static view of class; which ignores the subjective processes involved in becoming a class, and it is also crucial, as his book points out, to recognise that the question of the construction of identity, individually and collectively, cannot simply be read off capitalist productive relations. This is why I have counterposed Paul Gilroy to Peter Leonard at this point. However, it is important not to make an equally unfortunate mistake which involves appearing to write off the working class altogether, via an unproblematical reliance on Gorz (1982), who suggests of the working class that it is a class 'whose interests, capacities and skills are functional to the existing productive forces, which themselves are functional solely to the rationality of capital' (p. 68). It appears that Gorz, in pursuit of the libertarian project of the abolition of work, is perhaps tempted to overstate the extent to which this is already taking place.

A declining workforce may nevertheless increase production. There may also be increases in levels of white-collar trade unionism, and even of militancy within that sector. Reorganising and restructuring, or relocating a workforce is not the same thing as abolishing it, or its potential power, and the fact that workers in a particular industry, or country, may be disinclined to use the power that having an important place in production and being numerically stronger than their employers gives them, is not the same thing as this power's disappearing forever.

An empirical investigation of current structural change in the British economy is attempted by Callinicos and Harman (1987). It appears that there is little evidence for the more extreme versions of structural change, of which Gorz (1982) is, in my view, an example (see also Callinicos 1989: 122; Milliband 1989: 45, 49 and 50; Sivanandan 1990: 19–58; Wood 1986: 15–18 and 72).

A multiplicity of sites of power and resistance to power

Perhaps Foucault (1984) has a point when he suggests that power always produces resistance. For Foucault there is a multiplicity of diffuse powers. He suggests that 'power is everywhere; not because it embraces everything, but because it comes from everywhere' (p. 93), therefore there can be no 'single locus of great Refusal, no soul of revolt, source of all rebellions, or pure law of the revolutionary' (p. 96).

This position differs from that of Gilroy, in that there is no single revolutionary agent, whether it be the proletariat, black resistance, or the otherwise disadvantaged or dispossessed. For Foucault if revolution happens at all, it will be as a result of the many resistances breaking through the power that has produced them.

There are social-work texts which attempt to offer a social-work practice that endeavours to be anti-racist, and Lena Dominelli (1988) in *Anti-Racist Social Work* offers a list of 10 changes in social work which need to be made to make anti-racist social work firmly implanted. They are worth considering in full. She argues that it is necessary to

- Change the current definition of the social work task to one which does not render oppression invisible;
- Negate the 'objectivity' currently imbedded in a professionalism underpinning a status quo which has been seriously wanting;
- Alter the existing power relations between the users of services and workers. The voice of the 'expert' should not substitute for that of the oppressed;
- Not deny the consumers their right to determine the types of welfare provision on offer;

- Stop treating people's welfare at both individual and group level as a commodity that can be rationed for the purposes of controlling people and their aspirations. Instead, it should enhance personal fulfilment and wellbeing;
- Change the basis of training which assumes a false neutrality on the major social and ethical issues of the day to one making explicit its value base and taking a moral and political stance against oppression in any of its forms;
- Terminate an allocation of power and resources perpetuating injustice and misery and replace it with one committed to implementing justice and equality for all;
- End the theoretical separation between social work and a) other key elements of the state, especially welfare sections, e.g. housing... and b) the law and order apparatus including the police and the courts, the Home Office and the Immigration Service. Instead, the connections between each of these parts must be made visible;
- End the separation between policy and practice, exposing the connections between them; and
- Replace the lack of political commitment to end racial inequality, with one operating in the opposite direction.

(p. 163)

Dominelli adds that

From the variety of changes that are envisaged, it is clear that not only will anti-racist social work end racism but it will expose and tackle other forms of oppression which are reproduced by and perpetuated through social work too.

(p. 163)

There are three questions which all of this immediately begs. The first one concerns the tall order involved in expecting social work to end racism. This is desirable, but if it is achievable it cannot be achieved via social work alone, whatever changes it may make. This implied view of the matter risks producing a new professionalism, in place of the old criticised one, that now becomes expert in the elimination of racism, and which, whatever the intention might be, also risks imposing its own view or version of anti-racism upon black people, by casting them in the role of always and everywhere a victim (see Gilroy 1987: 11). While this is not Lena Dominelli's intention, especially given the changes she wishes to see, there remains a risk of this sort of reading.

Anti-racism and a critique of equal-opportunities policies

Of course it is essential that equal-opportunities policies be supported, demanded and developed where there are none, or no adequate implementation of them. Nevertheless there is a danger of relying simply and solely upon this as a strategy. Though Lena Dominelli makes reference in her text to Paul Gilroy (1987) she does not appear to take up the criticisms of existing antiracist strategies that he offers. For instance, Gilroy (1987) points out that

> If, as has been suggested, the 'race' issue has been seen from the vantage point of a sympathetic liberalism as a matter of policy rather than politics... the tasks of a more sustained and thoroughgoing anti-racism must include an attempt to show how the administration of institutional reforms... can be articulated to a sound grasp of extra-institutional policies.

The problem involved in these sorts of strategies for Paul Gilroy is that they run the risk of confining racism and anti-racism to institutional settings. Anti-racist strategies, if they are to be 'credible outside the institutional setting in which they were dreamed up' should not 'have the effect of appearing to reduce the complexity of black life to an effect of racism' (Gilroy 1987: 150). He sees a danger in presenting racism as simply a struggle between 'victims and perpetrators'. This evacuates black people from history, that is, their own history of struggle and resistance, not recognising them as 'actors capable of making complex choices in the furtherance of their own liberation' (p. 150).

It does seem to me that these dangers are present in the strategy offered by Lena Dominelli. However, it is also important to remember that as one strategy among many potential and actual ones, both in institutional, and extra-institutional settings, it is an important one and should be supported, albeit critically and with a clear idea of its limitations. After all it is only after the experience, for instance, of municipal anti-racism, that a critique of it can be fully developed.

Feminist social work

There are also texts available which offer a particular focus on social work in the context of gender. Dominelli and McCleod (1989), *Feminist Social Work*, is one such example. Feminism, they suggest, involves an egalitarian stance and therefore the authors oppose other social divisions which involve dominance and subordination.

In the context of this book, which is concerned with the dilemmas that social workers working with children and families face, the chapter concerning statutory social work is of particular interest and therefore the focus is mainly on that chapter. The authors suggest that

> Feminist initiatives have begun to make inroads into a fourth dimension of practice – statutory social work. In analysing the significance and potential of this work, we discuss the contribution made to feminist analysis by radical and Marxist critiques of statutory social work's social control role, as the precursors of a feminist approach.
>
> (p. 101)

The chapter then considers in more detail many of the texts reviewed earlier. As well as concluding, as one might expect, that Marxist texts do not integrate an account of gender centrally into their analysis, they conclude that

> By consigning statutory social work to reinforcing middle-class ideology and agency norms, a Marxist approach fails to develop forms of social work practice which incorporate sensitive work at an individual level, take account of both personal experience and broader social conditions, respond to grass roots activism, utilize the resources of local and central bureaucracies in the pursuit of egalitarian aims...
>
> (p. 106)

The authors take the view that the tension and difficulty surrounding a theoretical analysis of class and gender is 'still in the grip of adding an analysis of gender onto or into a class analysis of oppression and worrying about which should take precedence in the process' (p. 106).

There are difficult questions of emphasis in this sort of analysis and one would expect feminist social work to place particular emphasis on gender. However, if a hierarchy of oppressions is to be avoided, then a reading should also be avoided in which social divisions are always seen as vertical – for example, male, female, black, white, lesbian/gay, heterosexual, people with a disability, able-bodied, and no doubt many more – and rarely horizontal, for example, class, occupation etc. Otherwise class in its objective economic context, with the attendant social stratification, would only appear as an absence. This risks in turn leaving the work vulnerable to a crude reading in which a person's position in the vertical division of the social order is seen as all-determining, which of course it is not. Sivanandan (1990) points out that

> The touchstone of any issue-based or identity-based politics has to be the lowest common denominator in our society. A women's movement that does not derive its politics from the needs, freedoms, rights of the most disadvantaged among them is by that very token reformist and elitist. Conversely a politics that is based on women qua women is inward looking and narrow and nationalist and, above all, failing of its own experience. So too, the blacks or gays or whoever. So too, are the green and peace movements Eurocentric and elitist that do not derive their politics from the most ecologically devastated and war ravaged parts of the world. Class cannot just be a matter for identity, it has to be the focus of commitment.
>
> (p. 44)

The chapter commences with a critique of existing statutory social work; feminist social work, it suggests, 'proceeds from a critique of its social control role' (p. 107). The predominance of women as clients, carers, and as social workers (usually and overwhelmingly in lower grades than men) is the starting point. The authors suggest that 'the policy of community care, that is, of care centred within families as opposed to institutional provision should be decoded as "care by women who bear the main responsibility for it" ' (p. 111).

Feminist social work and social control

Dominelli and McCleod recognise that it is 'not an exaggeration to describe the characteristic and most high profile' statutory service 'at present as the pursuit and surveillance of parental failure' (1989: 111). However, they do not wish to give a reader the impression that 'feminism is resistant to any controls being placed on individuals' behaviour' (p. 112). By way of illustration they contrast a feminist approach's considering separating a sexually abused child from her male abuser, to a more 'liberal' family-therapy approach which may endeavour to keep the family together. On the other hand they point out that a feminist approach to the question of social control does not entail social workers' 'taking the part of a woman over and above the interests of others' (p. 112). They make the point that the rights of children and mothers may conflict, in terms of the child's right to physical and emotional well-being.

However, the authors explicitly resist placing the interests of the child above that of the mother. Even where it is necessary to separate a mother from her children, then in doing this the social worker would be engaging in protecting the interests of the children whilst at the same time trying to convey to the mother that her behaviour without condoning it is not reflective of her own individual pathology...but rather sadly indicative of social relations prevailing more generally in respect of parents and children...At the same time it is incumbent on feminist social workers to convey the same messages to their agency and beyond (p. 113).

There is a very serious problem involved in this. It is quite simply the fact that if child abuse is always and everywhere 'indicative of prevailing social relations', then since these social relations prevail everywhere, so should child abuse, and of course it doesn't. This passage gives the impression that there is never individual pathology in the world, only oppressive social relations. Whilst not denying that oppressive social relations can have, and frequently do have, unpleasant consequences, any individual explanation ought not to be discounted in advance. If it were, social workers would be at a loss to explain why many people, indeed the majority of people in oppressive social conditions, or social relationships, or occupying social divisions in society which may and do involve oppression, nevertheless bring up their children without abusing them.

This earlier passage is reductionist, it contains the implicit promise that if oppressive social relationships can be dispensed with, then so can child abuse. But this is only true if there is a direct one-to-one causal relationship between oppressed parents and abused children, which, quite simply, there is not. Social workers conveying this message to their 'agencies and beyond' would run the risk of ridicule. The task itself is not criticised, nor is its emergence as a central task for social workers traced historically; it is simply implied that a feminist social worker will accomplish the task more effectively because she better understands its causes.

Having said this, the book is a serious attempt to outline a potential social-work practice based on feminist understandings and is therefore of real use. However, it has similar gaps and silences in relation to class that the literature it criticises has in terms of gender, and it is possible, if it is read literally, that it may only exchange a crudeness about class for an equal crudeness in relation to gender.

Women-centred practice

Hanmer and Stathem (1988) (*Women and Social Work – Towards a Women Centred Practice*) offer an analysis of women and social work which has a 'primary intention' and an 'ultimate aim' (p. 3). Their primary intention is to 'make women visible as clients and as workers' (p. 3). Their ultimate aim is 'to facilitate assessment and planning so that non-sexist practice can emerge' (pp. 3–4).

The book is explicitly confined to social work and is, therefore, in an important sense less generally programmatic than much of the literature reviewed earlier. The practice is not, for instance, linked to a process of more general transformation in social relations. The aim is more modest. It is an attempt to 'weave together a women-centred perspective on women, both as clients and as workers, with suggestions on how to begin to realise women-centred practice'(p. 4).

The first chapter of the book focuses upon both commonalities and diversities between clients and women social workers and it opens with definitions of both sexism and racism. Racism, they suggest, is

> The belief in the inherent superiority of one race over all others and thereby the right to dominance. Sexism, the belief in the inherent superiority of one sex over the other and thereby the right to dominance.
>
> (p. 7)

The definitions of any form of oppression play a crucial role in developing any political practice, inclusive of social-work practice, based upon them, and should therefore be critically scrutinised. There are problems with these definitions. All appear to confine the problems to belief, and to prejudice, and in addition the definition of racism appears to make the concepts of race and sex categories of equal certainty. Clearly, however they are not sex is biological, though gender is socially constructed; race, however, is not simply or even mainly biological. To the list of authors so far quoted in this chapter who have relevantly criticised the types of definition that appear in the work quoted earlier, for example, Sivanandan (1990), Gilroy (1987), could be added Smith (1989). She suggests that 'the erroneous belief that human races exist as distinct biological types, identified by physical traits and reflected in cultural diversity, has longstanding, widespread and disturbingly enduring appeal' (Smith 1989: 2).

There is a danger in the definition of racism offered above of unconsciously perpetuating this erroneous belief. At the same time, however, it is important to avoid depriving people of a subjective collective identity, via which, at crucial points, they may live their lives, and collectively resist oppression. Nevertheless, it is important to explicitly contradict the idea of race as biological certainty because otherwise a myth may well be perpetuated via an uncritical reading of the text of the definition.

In fairness to these authors, however, it should be remembered that they attempt to focus on both commonality and difference in relation to women as workers and clients. It should also be remembered that the attempt to apply political theory will always leave a tension between elaborate and fully refined theory on the one hand, and the practice that is based upon it on the other.

In the chapter entitled 'Women as Carers' the authors (Hanmer and Stathem 1988) provide a section concerning the concept of 'fit mothering'. They argue that motherhood is 'becoming more tightly structured' (p. 56) via the concept of the 'fit mother' which is itself being 'more tightly defined'(p. 56). They make the point that mothers are monitored by doctors, social workers, health visitors etc. It is also pointed out that courts may make judgements about the fitness of a mother as part and parcel of a judgement where a woman has committed an offence. It could be added that this judgement is also made when an offence, for example, domestic violence, and even rape, have been committed against a woman. They add that there is no similar concept of a 'fit father'. The consequence is that social workers will often focus all of their attention on a woman in a household, even where there is a man with parental responsibility, or otherwise in the role of caring for a child. This is important and may in itself have contributed to tragic outcomes in social work with children. One such example is the Maria Colwell case which is considered in detail in Chapter 7 of this book.

The authors do not consider the question of child abuse in any degree of detail, though they do make the point that within the context of an increased interest in sexual abuse, in which the perpetrators are overwhelmingly men, the concept of 'fit mothering' hardly applies, and the absence of a concept of 'fit father' raises the need to examine these assumptions.

The work in total is more measured, and yet more limited than the work of Dominelli and McCleod (1989) or Dominelli (1988). It is more limited because its focus is entirely on the social work as an activity in itself. In other words while it is programmatic, the programme is for social work in and of itself, unlike the authors cited immediately above; and unlike the Marxist literature also reviewed, it does not see the transformation of social work, via the practice it envisages, as an explicit part of a process of wider change within the social order. It is more measured in the sense that it is less rhetorical and, for example, while it is keen to separate 'individual responsibility from the social and economic context in which women live' (p. 142), it nevertheless explicitly recognises the multifaceted nature of any work which may be involved in helping to relieve individual distress.

The book of course suffers from its limitation; for instance much of the critiqué that Gilroy (1987) offers of municipal anti-racism could be levelled at these authors and indeed most of the others that are reviewed earlier and who attempt to focus on gender or race. We can be left with a situation in which the worst aspects of oppression, be they racist, sexist, heterosexist or anti-working class, are untouched simply because they take place outside an institutional context, that is, on the streets, in the home, on a picket line etc. On the other hand, its more limited and consequently more modest focus does not lead itinto the trap of the over-promising, for example, bringing an end to racism, implicit in Dominelli (1988), and it enables the authors to focus more clearly on a potentially positive practice.

It is important to remember that the idea of a non-sexist social-work practice in a society that remains sexist is something of a tall order, and also that the definitions of oppressions that the authors offer, though not always the practice, run the risk of substituting fragmentation and division for reductionism and homogenisation. There is also the problem of the reduction of class to a question of identity and prejudice, via the concept of 'classism'. There is surely more to be said about class oppression than the issue of prejudice, and if some Marxisms have been overarching in their analysis of class, then it is not a sufficient response to strip it of all structural understanding, and thereby forget that the question of exploitation of working-class people's labour, be they women, men, black, gay, lesbian, heterosexual, or people with or without physical disabilities, or learning difficulties, is a central feature of the society in which we live.

Radical social work today

Langan and Lee (1989) edit a volume entitled *Radical Social Work Today*. It is a collection of 15 essays written by social-work academics, social and community work practitioners, researchers and development officers. There are articles ranging from a retrospective analysis of the contribution of radical social work, to issues in relation to social work and unemployment, developments within social service departments, inclusive of the decentralisation debate, feminism, gender and social work, violence and the emergence of the concept of dangerousness, black politics in social work, black women and radical social work, radical social work with older people, residential care, community work in a recession, black perspectives in social work and radical probation work. The essay entitled 'Whatever Happened to Radical Social Work?' is of particular historical interest since it attempts to trace the impact that the 'movement' associated with the body of literature reviewed earlier has had upon contemporary social work.

The authors point out that the radical social work 'movement' widened the scope of modern social work (p. 2). By this they mean that it 'introduced a wider set of issues and put politics on the agenda'. The last 15 years have, say the authors, however, fundamentally changed the context in which social work operates (p. 2). They are able to identify four factors in this new climate affecting social work. The first factor is 15 years, with ups and downs, of economic recession and a Conservative government, both of which have increased the workload of social workers, via austerity policies, community-care policies, and the pressure upon mainly women carers that they bring about. Grouped within this particular factor the authors include the suggestion that 'national panics about child abuse and crime have resulted in a heavier burden of work for social workers' (p. 2).

While increased concern about child abuse may well have increased social workers' workloads, the suggestion that this is explicable simply and solely via recourse to a moral panic can be criticised. Chapter 7 of this book offers an analysis of the concept of moral panic in relation to child abuse and of the discourse contained in the *Report of the Committee of Inquiry into the Care and Supervision Provided in Relation to Maria Colwell* (DHSS 1974), and its impact upon the formation of the 1975 Children Act.

The second factor which has changed the context in which social work operates is 'the unprecedented barrage of public criticism and condemnation' (see pp. 2–3). The authors note a paradox concerning the media reaction to questions of child sexual abuse, in which the notion of the radical social worker as an 'ineffectual liberal' was exchanged for that of the social worker as a 'zealot' (p. 3). However, they appear not to see that this has implications for the concept that a 'scare' or 'moral panic' in relation to child abuse was simply and solely the determining factor in relation to all of this condemnation in the first place, since it is difficult for a notion of 'moral panic' among the public/media to explain a belief that social workers intervene both too little and too much. It is able to 'explain' the former but not the latter.

The third shift is concerned with 'the drive to press social workers into assuming a more coercive and interventionist role in policing deviant families in Thatcher's Britain' (p. 3).

The fourth shift has been well rehearsed earlier in the criticisms offered in relation to this body of literature. It concerns the fact that radical social work has been criticised by representatives of the oppressed. The point is made that 'it would be disingenuous to ignore the difficulties involved in trying to make the radical social work movement truly representative of and accountable to all sections of the oppressed' (p. 10). They nevertheless add that 'there is a danger that these tensions may lead to the increasing fragmentation of the radical movement' (p. 10).

The authors further suggest that the main weakness of radical social work was the fact that it had an 'underdeveloped political strategy' (p. 13), in that it found it difficult to translate socialist principles into concrete ways of helping people as a social work. Related to this is their view that early radical social work saw welfare as 'either functioning on behalf of capitalism, or as the product of working class struggle'. This is thought to lead to the problem that the left was dismissive of the 'reactionary aspects of state welfare'. Hence when welfare became an object of intervention for a right wing government, 'it found itself ill-prepared to defend its progressive features' (see p. 13).

This view, while broadly true, appears to over-homogenise 'the left' and radical social workers within it. It also risks giving the impression that 'the left' alone, outside a generalised and focused resistance much beyond itself, can in some way defend the 'progressive elements of welfare'. But surely the problem was that while there was and is resistance, it was and is insufficiently generalised, that is, widespread, and insufficiently focused, that is, specific. What determines the focus and degree of resistance is, to some extent, the question of the degree of popularity of that which requires defending. The less generally and genuinely popular it is, the less will be the extent of, and the less clear will be the focus of, resistance.

In terms of welfare, for instance, the strike by ambulance workers in the late 1980s was popular. The workers, though they did not win the strike, were well supported financially and in opinion polls, etc. This enabled them to hold out longer and avoid a humiliating defeat. The service that they provide is popular. The service that social workers provide, on the other hand, and in spite of the prefigurative endeavours of the radicals in their number, is not always popular, though there are examples of social workers organising with users to defend a genuinely popular service under threat. It is here that the concept of 'authoritarian populism' (Hall 1988: 41) can be of use, but of course it requires specificity, that is, in this particular case an understanding of why some aspects of welfare and people's experience of them are less contradictory, and therefore those aspects are more popular than others. Given genuine popularity, other issues come into focus, for example, opportunity, confidence and the assessment of the potential prospects for success, etc.

The article concludes by declaring that 'never has it been more important for social workers to act in ways that minimize the worst effects of current state policies and maximize the potential for resistance of the underclass' (p. 17). There is the assumption of an underclass here. But the concept is a complex and contested one. A number of questions could be raised, for example, is the underclass a permanent feature of contemporary capitalist society? Is its membership permanent? Who is in it? Does its population change: Is the formation of a class, even an underclass, merely a matter of objective circumstance or does it require in addition a subjective forming? How many people would identify themselves as 'underclass'? These difficulties are best acknowledged, if an inexperienced reader is not to take an author's assertion for the truth. There would remain, the question of the power of the underclass, and its sectional nature, etc.; for instance, it is hard to imagine what a 'common political programme' might be in this context. Notwithstanding the criticisms made earlier of this article, the article itself and the collection of essays in the book offer a serious attempt to overcome the limitation of some of the earlier work.

In considering the body of literature cited earlier, assessments have been made specifically in relation to each particular text. In summary, however, the following criticisms at a more general level can be made.

There is a tendency in many of the texts to assert and assume rather than to argue. In addition there is a tendency at times to be formulaic and reductionist, and as a result to over-promise, particularly in the context of a limited political strategy and a limited degree of developed social-work practice.

There is insufficient discussion about competing definitions of various forms of oppression. This risks a crude reading where the one definition provided is read as the truth of the matter. There is a permanent tension between, on the one hand, reductionism and homogenisation, and on the other hand, diversity and fragmentation. This is sometimes because of the difficulties in dealing with complex questions of emphasis, and because of the genuine difficulty involved in attempting to provide a general theory which does not reduce, or appear to reduce, all other oppressions to an effect of any particular one of them.

A further problem is that, in the main, there is insufficient attention in this literature to the attempt to understand individuals as individuals, not simply in the context of the discipline of psychology but also in terms of the kind of sociology that concerns itself with individuals.

In particular relation to statutory social work – and to working with children and families in that context, which involves necessarily a focus upon child protection, etc. – these texts are particularly weak. Few of them devote much attention to the problem, and those of them that do attend to it do not consider in detail or in depth the historical emergence of this particular and increasingly central task. What all of this lacks, in relation to this issue, is an appropriate degree of empirical specificity. This is an important problem because these texts are the only widely available, specifically social-work texts which claim to offer any historical account of the emergence of contemporary social-work practice. They are, or have been, influential in the field. It is this problem that has prompted a consideration of whether elements of discourse analysis may be useful in developing a fuller account.

There is a tension between discourse analysis and Marxism, in that the former tends to be more Foucauldian in its approach. This tension, and an endeavour to explore and negotiate it, constitutes the subject material of Chapter 2.

Chapter 2

Questions of theory

DISCOURSE ANALYSIS AND SOCIAL WORK

Rojek *et al.* (1988), *Social Work and Received Ideas* – seeks to apply discourse analysis to social work, and therefore this chapter will first briefly consider that text. It will argue that it offers a crude version of both Marxism and the various strands of feminism, to which it is in part a critical response. The chapter will also argue that the particular version of social work, which is termed 'Subjectless social work', and the view of discourse analysis upon which it is based, also have a strong tendency to reductionism.

The authors suggest that 'the central argument of this book is that the language which social workers are trained to use in order to free clients very often has the effect of imprisoning them anew' (p. 1). They also indicate that their work is a critical response to both traditional social work and radical social work. While they recognise that there is complexity in classifying together very differing approaches under only two headings, in the context of those classified under 'traditional' they feel that, nevertheless, 'what unites [them] all is the aim of bringing about the adjustment of the client to presently existing conditions in society. Traditional social work is therefore about the technical management of personal problems and the maintenance of order' (p. 1). In terms of the classification 'radical' they feel that there are two common features to these diverse strands: all of them criticise traditional social work on the basis that it '(a) applies an ahistorical view of social work values, and (b) neglects to itemise the structural context in which personal problems are produced and reproduced' (p. 2).

The authors argue for a view of social work that is both dialectical and realist. They inform a reader that 'by dialectical we mean a view of social work which recognises that all things exist in time, and because of this they are contradictory, transient and changeable' (p. 2). This view of the notion of dialectical owes very little to Hegel or to Marx. Change for Hegel and Marx was not simply the commonplace assumption that because of time, all things are transient.

The authors further inform their readers that they

> use the term realism to refer to the view that a real, objective world exists independently of consciousness, which is however ascertainable by consciousness. We include nature, history and society in our notion of the real world. Our argument is that the conduct of individuals cannot be understood accurately unless it is placed in the context of natural, historical, and social relations.
>
> (p. 2)

However, there is, they say, a routine objection to realist theory, which is that it produces an overdeterministic model of human behaviour. Hence, realist theory, they suggest, is accused of supporting a passive view of human relations. They then suggest that this criticism 'certainly applied to both traditional and radical versions of realism in social work' (p. 3). It is said to apply in traditional social work because 'in particular angry and negative feelings are seen as abnormalities that threaten the social order. The notion that these feelings represent accurate and meaningful condemnations of deadening social relations is never seriously developed' (pp. 3–4). The authors offer no source for this observation, and it is not a view that would be endorsed by many traditional social workers, certainly not from a casework perspective. A person may be invited to examine their anger or negative feelings, and in social work influenced by Freudian theory there may be a consideration of transference and counter-transference: that is, the idea that the anger may be about something other than what the person initially thinks it is. Alternatively a caseworker may take the view that anger and hostility is a positive force if they believe that it has previously been sublimated. Whatever view is taken of a particular anger, a caseworker would rarely, if they were attempting serious casework, start from the premise that all anger and hostility was bad because it threatened the social order.

Discourse theory and feminist social work

In relation to feminist endeavours, the authors suggest that while feminist approaches offer a potentially powerful approach to analysing social-work practice, nevertheless feminism offers a flawed approach. This is because 'feminism is ambiguous; it means very different things to different people . . . . In particular it assumes a unanimity on the subject – women's oppression – which does not exist' (Rojeck *et al.* 1988: 113).

It is not clear from their text what they feel is wrong with the fact that feminism is not unanimous in its approach. It is not clear either that feminism does assume unanimity on the subject of women's oppression. The authors do not quote a source for this observation. Indeed they make the observation after having reviewed three competing views within feminist theory of the oppression of women: those of liberal feminism, radical separatism and Marxist feminism. It appears that they see unanimity where there is none, and yet nevertheless criticise diversity because it isn't unanimous. They do not offer a response to the potential rejoinder from a feminist of any perspective that in the diversity of feminist theory there exists a strength and not a weakness.

Discourse theory and the critique of radical social work

The authors criticise radical social work and offer the view that

> Radical social work operated with a one sided view of power. Indeed, power was equated with control. For example the standard criticism of traditional social work was that it simply functioned to control the client and block progressive change.
>
> (Rojeck *et al.* 1988: 37)

Once again, the authors do not quote a source for this observation, and in the radical social-work literature reviewed in Chapter 1 of this book no text offered that view. Indeed even in the very earliest radical social-work text, that is, Bailey and Brake (1975), Peter Leonard suggests that

> To see social workers, in short, as *simply* the willing henchmen of the ruling class in its exercise of social control is to take an undialectical view. It overestimates the rationality and monolithic nature of the capitalist state in its ability to determine in detail the activities of an occupation.
>
> (Leonard 1975: 49)

When (Rojeck *et al.* 1988) turn specifically to their chapter on discourse analysis and social work, they indicate that they reject the humanist idea that human beings share core essential features. They suggest that

> Notions of common 'consciousness', 'reason', 'compassion', 'freedom' and 'choice', it is said, are merely expressions of humanist ideology, i.e. they refer to a mythical rather than a real state of affairs. Moreover the radical positions of Marxism and feminism in social work and elsewhere are faulted on the grounds that they reproduce the basic assumptions of orthodox humanism.
>
> (Rojeck *et al.* 1988: 117)

The implications for social work of discourse analysis

Discourse analysis, they suggest, raises important points for social work, and they list four of them. Discourse analysis, they say, shows that there is nothing fundamental or inevitable about the form of social work. The second point that they make is that discourse analysis reverses the accepted notion of need in humanist social work. This is because

> Humanist social work portrays the social worker as the servant of needs which spread out from the client (the subject). We have referred to these needs on several occasions in this book. Among the most prominent are the needs for compassion, respect, dignity and trust. Social work, the humanists say, is about fulfilling these needs through the provision of care with responsibility. Yet, from the perspective of discourse analysis, this puts the cart before the horse. Compassion, respect, dignity, etc., do not arise spontaneously from the client. Rather they are constructed through discourse and the client is expected to fit in with them.
>
> (p. 31)

There is a risk of a reader taking the above too literally and the consequence of so doing would be simply that one should abandon these values and recognise them as the discursive construction that they are said here to be. A philosophy of social work which risks relegating compassion, respect and dignity to the status of a discursive construction, it could be argued, is in the end unethical.

However, the objection to the above is not simply ethical. It also seems that the position above runs the risk, if it is taken too literally, of becoming absurd. For instance, social workers are confronted with situations that make them feel compassionate towards the people facing them. Just one simple example would be of a woman who had burned down her flat in an episode of extreme depression/distress/illness, and after a brief spell in a mental hospital was discharged to that same flat in the condition in which she left it. There is a risk here of imagining that any compassionate endeavours, for, with and on behalf of this woman, constituted only a discursive construction which she was required to fit into. This risks giving discourse an all-embracing power which, as far as I am able to see, reproduces what these authors wish to avoid, that is, social theory which offers a passive view of social relations.

It is often the case that the, relatively speaking, powerless people who are the subjects and object of social-work intervention would receive no help at all were it not for the compassion of others. Hence, it seems to me to be important to avoid the risk of embracing a theory which can be read, albeit crudely, as minimising such compassion.

What the paragraph quoted earlier lacks is any degree of the dialectical understanding which these authors nevertheless suggest actually informs their work. It is one thing for a discourse to be suspect, to be contaminated with power/knowledge and to mobilise concepts such as compassion, truth, dignity, respect etc., in its project, and in that process, in part, to mould, construct, reconstruct and manipulate these qualities. I do not doubt that this takes place; indeed in the analysis of the discourses under consideration in this book some of this will be seen. However, this is not the same thing as denying the reality, outside discourse, of these qualities.

To paraphrase Leonard (1975), quoted earlier, and to change the alleged determining agent, it could be suggested that to see social workers, in short, as simply the willing henchpeople of the ruling discourse is to take an undialectical view. It overestimates the rationality and monolithic nature of the discourse in its ability to determine in detail the activities of an occupation, and its subjects/objects of intervention. If the transparent reduction of complex multiple causes to a singular simplistic economic cause is called economism, then perhaps the same mistake with discourse as the simple singular cause can best be termed discourseism. Needless to say it is equally flawed.

For all the endeavours in the text to overcome the 'routine objection' to realist theory, which is that it produces an 'overdeterministic model of human behaviour', and stands accused of 'endorsing a passive view of human relations' (see earlier), it appears that in fact the authors themselves produce a theory which can be objected to on the same grounds.

Discourse analysis and the possibility of knowledge

The third issue which the authors suggest that discourse analysis raises is the fact that discourse theory is 'iconoclastic' in that it 'calls into question not only the meaning of social work knowledge, but even the possibility of such knowledge' (Rojek *et al.* 1988: 132). This sits uneasily with a commitment to the kind of realism that they explicitly endorse. The authors leave themselves open to the routine objection that can be levelled against all those who deny the possibility of knowledge: that is, how do they know, since knowing is explicitly ruled out by their own theory because

> There is no privileged or objective meaning, because there is no privileged or objective knowledge. It follows that humanist social work is doubly damned. To begin with it is said to base itself in a sphere of 'reality' which does not exist, i.e. common human needs … In the second place its claim that social work knowledge is more detached, objective and truthful than other forms of knowledge is rejected as indefensible. The social worker is trapped in the restless play of language and other sign systems as are all other people. *There is no escape.*
>
> (p. 132, my emphasis)

It may be the case that, sometimes, some social-work knowledge over-claims on its own behalf. But this is not the same as the suggestion that there can be no knowledge because we are all trapped within the restless play of language. It would also be an obligation upon authors taking this position to explain how they themselves had 'escaped', when they have asserted that escape is impossible. It is hard to resist the conclusion that these authors want to claim knowledge while simultaneously denying its possibility.

Discourse analysis and relations of power

The fourth implication of discourse analysis for social work, it is claimed, is that social-work relations need to be considered as relations of power. Social work, they suggest, aims to normalise social relations by rooting out 'deviance', 'antagonism', and 'pathology'. However, social work has not been successful, because clients 'in need' still exist. The authors do not provide an explanation of what is meant by 'need' in this context, since they cannot mean it in the alleged 'ideological' humanist context. They add that for Foucault and 'other writers on discourse theory', it has nevertheless been 'spectacularly successful' in 'another latent goal of the system', that is, 'the deliberate production of the pathologised personality' (see p. 132). They add that 'from the perspective of discourse analysis the social work discourse, (a) creates abnormality, by specifying the nature of the pathological, and (b) imposes solutions on the client by its access to the institutions of discipline, punishment and moral regulation' (pp. 132–3).

Humanism as the doxa of social work

The authors conclude their chapter with a definition of the term 'doxa'. They suggest that it 'is used in discourse analysis to refer to the prevailing view of things, which very often prevails to the extent that people are unaware that it is only one of several possible alternative views' (p. 143). They add that 'We have argued that the doxa of social work is humanism' (p. 143), and that 'Discourse analysis is concerned, among other things, with unravelling the veil of doxa and awakening the sleeper from sleep' (p. 143). In conclusion the authors quote Foucault (1981: 13), in suggesting that discourse analysis seeks to avoid the conclusion

> That this then is what needs to be done. It should be an instrument for those who fight, those who resist and refuse what is. Its use should be in the process of conflict and confrontation, essays in refusal. It doesn't have to lay down the law. It isn't a stage in programming. It is a challenge to what is.
>
> (Foucault 1981: 145)

In considering the earlier text a number of criticisms have been offered. To briefly summarise, it appears that the authors attempt to establish their own position at the expense of, at times, adopting a crude version of the positions which they seek to transcend. Nevertheless, in doing so it appears that they themselves become immersed in the theoretical difficulties that they claim exist in the literature that they criticise. It appears that they grant too much determining power to discourse and consequently insufficient power to its subjects and objects, in spite of their desire and commitment to do the contrary. They appear to write off the possibility of knowledge altogether, and also the utility of reason, even of a criticised reason, even though they appear themselves to make truth claims, based on reasoned argument. This is therefore not an adequate foundation for either a social work based upon discourse theory, or an adequate theoretical method through which to analyse discourse. Though, for instance, the radical social-work literature was criticised in Chapter 1 of this book for reductionism, the level of crude determinism that these authors attribute to it is not sustainable if a fair reading of the literature is undertaken.

It is also the case that the crude determinism that may sometimes exist, though unevenly, in the radical social-work literature cannot be read simply as a result of its debt to Marx. In order to establish that proposition it would first be necessary to establish that Marx was *himself reductionist*. In addition to this, discourse analysis has no need either to abolish the subjects of the analysed discourse and turn them into passive objects. In fact, it is often this discursive move that I attempt to uncover and expose, and strongly criticise within the discourse considered in the rest of this book. There is all the difference in the world between history as a process without a collective subject, and without a guarantee of a happy (revolutionary) ending, and life without the existence of active, conscious, individual subjects capable of transcending their current state of consciousness. The authors under consideration seem to slide from the need to avoid the former, into the entirely unnecessary abolition of the latter.

The work of Foucault, especially his later work, indicates that he himself did not have such a deterministic and passive role for the individual subject. Hence it is necessary to outline the ways in which a non-reductionist version of the work of Foucault can be of utility in the project of discourse analysis.

Power/knowledge

For Foucault, the definition of the *dispositif*, or apparatus, is as a 'thoroughly heterogeneous ensemble consisting of discourses, institutions, architectural forms, regulatory decisions, laws, administrative measures, scientific statements, philosophical, moral and philanthropic propositions – in short, the said and the unsaid' (Foucault 1980: 194). His interests therefore do not simply concern language, or even discourse. Both the said and the unsaid, that is, the discursive and the non-discursive, are of importance. Hence it is not the case for Foucault, unlike the post-structuralist thinkers with which he is sometimes linked, that there is no escape from language because it has no 'outside'.

Foucault is more worldly than this. His interest is in power and knowledge, and the ways in which people are constituted as subjects through power and knowledge. He believes that 'one's point of reference should not be the great model of language and signs, but that of war and battle...relations of power, not relations of meaning' (Foucault 1980: 114).

He is, suspicious of truth claims in themselves. This is because, for him, they form a central part of the technique of discourse. They are a chain that links the subjects and objects of a discourse to that discourse.

Relativism and the critique of the concept of ideology

This radical relativism has led Foucault to the conclusion that ideology is a concept that cannot be used without circumspection. The reasons for this are threefold. He suggests that

> Like it or not, it always stands in opposition to something else that is supposed to count as truth... The second drawback is that the concept of ideology refers, I think necessarily, to something of the order of a subject. Thirdly ideology stands in a secondary position relative to something which functions as its infrastructure, as its material, economic determinant.
>
> (Foucault 1980: 118)

Foucault therefore does not attempt to analyse ideology. This would grant too much status to the particular discourse of Marxism. He is interested in the analysis of *all* discourse. In his approach to analysing discourse he does not

> Question the discourses for their silent meanings but on the fact and conditions of their manifest appearance; not on the contents which they may conceal, but on the transformations they may have effectuated; not on the meaning which is maintained in them like a perpetual origin, but on the field where they coexist, remain and disappear. It is a question of the analysis of the discourses in their exterior dimensions. From which arise three consequences:
>
> 1) Treat past discourse not as a theme for commentary which would revive it, but as a monument to be described in its character disposition.
> 2) Seek in the discourse not its laws of construction, as do the structural methods, but its conditions of existence.
> 3) Refer the discourse not to the thought, to the mind or to the subject which might have given rise to it, but to the practical field in which it is deployed.
>
> (Foucault 1978: 15)

Discourse as a regime of truth

A discourse can be seen as a regime of truth operating through a set of organising rules or principles, which allow the possibility of true and false statements. The organising rules or principles are independent of the statements made in any particular discourse. Discourse therefore makes possible a field of knowledge. It is this process which Foucault wishes to analyse in the particular way outlined above, since, for Foucault, 'truth is linked by a circular relation to systems of power which produce it and sustain it, and to effects of power which it induces and which redirect it, a regime of truth' (Foucault 1977).

For Foucault all of this is linked to the question of subjectivity, and it is this question which he has said has motivated his entire project. He clearly informs his readers that he would 'like to say, first of all, what has been the goal of my work during the last twenty years. It has not been to analyse the phenomena of power, nor to elaborate the foundations of such an analysis' (Foucault 1982: 208). His objective 'instead, has been to create a history of the different modes by which, in our culture, human beings are made subjects' (Foucault 1982: 208).

In this process he has isolated three 'modes of objectification' which are

a. the modes of inquiry which try to give themselves the status of science,

b. what I shall call 'dividing practices' (by which the subject is either divided in her or himself or divided from others, e.g. the mad and the sane, the sick and the healthy), and

c. the way a human being turns him or herself into a subject. For example . . . how men have learned to recognise themselves as subjects of 'sexuality'.

(Foucault 1982: 208)

Foucault points out that the state is implicated in these processes of objectification. The modern state, he suggests, did not develop above individuals

ignoring what they are and even their very existence, but on the contrary, as a very sophisticated structure, in which individuals can be integrated, under one condition; that this individuality would be shaped in a new form, and submitted, to a set of very specific patterns.

(Foucault 1982: 214)

He suggests that the state can be seen as a 'modern matrix of individualization', or a new form of pastoral power. This new form of pastoral power, however, does not have the traditional concerns of pastoral power, for it is concerned with our 'salvation' in this world, and not in the next. By 'salvation' he means, among other things, health, well-being, security, protection against accidents and so forth. In other words, he means 'a series of worldly aims' (Foucault 1982: 215).

Consequently the agents and officials of pastoral power have greatly increased. Sometimes they are located in the state apparatus, other times in private ventures, welfare societies and so forth. In addition, 'ancient institutions, for example the family, were also mobilised to take on pastoral functions' (Foucault 1982: 215). Pastoral power is also exercised by 'complex structures such as medicine... which also included public institutions such as hospitals' (Foucault 1982: 215).

The implication of this is quite simply that pastoral power, which for

> more than a millennium had been linked to a religious institution suddenly spread out into the whole social body; it found support in a whole number of institutions. And, instead of pastoral power and political power, more or less linked to each other, more or less rival, there was an individualizing 'tactic' which characterized a series of powers; those of the family, medicine, psychiatry, education, and employers.
>
> (Foucault 1982: 215)

This book owes a considerable debt to the work of Foucault. In the first place it is concerned with the analysis of the specific discourses contained in the various documents relating to British childcare legislation which it attempts to analyse, and Foucault properly points to the necessity of detailed empirical specificity and also to the issue of the diffuse nature of power, both of which are important in this context. Nevertheless, there are criticisms that can be made of his work, and it is important that attention be given to them since to do otherwise runs the risk of producing a skewed analysis of the issues under consideration.

A particular view of power

In an interview, late in his life, concerning his work *The History of Sexuality*, Foucault further elaborates his view of power. Indeed he indicates that the point of his project lies in the re-elaboration of the theory of power, because it has been 'too often reduced – following the model of juridical and philosophical thinking ... to the problem of sovereignty' (Foucault 1980: 187).

Perhaps the main reason for this is that he takes the view that the relationship between power and sex is not one merely of repression. This is because power is not simply a forbidding negation of desire. It is also creative – creative of categories (in this case) of sex and sexuality, creative of subjectivities, of subjects and of divisions within and between subjects etc.

A second important reason for this re-elaboration of the theory of power is the fact that Foucault himself admits that, in his work up to and including *Madness and Civilization* (1965), he himself had mistakenly seen power as an *essentially juridical mechanism*, that is, the law and its prohibitions, being at the centre of power. Foucault says of himself that he had 'too often' reduced power to these questions. However, he also implies that others have also made this reduction.

In the light of this it can fairly be asked; who is it really that has too often made this reduction? Whom can we find in the world who has consistently had a negative and never a positive conception of power? We could work by process of elimination. Not suffragettes, for instance, who demanded of 'power' that it give them the vote. Not philanthropic reformers who demanded of one power – the state – that it intervene into another power – that of the ownership of wealth – in order, for instance, to limit the length of the working day, or to ban the practice of sending children up chimneys in order to clean them, or to exclude children under certain ages from factory work etc. In short, it seems that history is littered with examples of people making both positive and negative demands upon power, power located in diffuse areas: for example, male power, state power, capitalist power etc.

The question could be put in a slightly different way. Who is it that too often reduces their thinking about power to the questions posed by the discourses of the political theorists of the sixteenth and seventeenth century, for example, Hobbes, Locke, Rousseau? It could be suggested that it would be hard to find such a person. However, if I try hard to imagine what such a person might 'look like', I would have to remember that a precondition for overestimating the importance of a particular discourse would at least be a great deal of familiarity with it, and involvement in it. It might be possible for such a person to overestimate the importance of the questions posed by such a discourse, even while rejecting some of the answers it provides. In the light of this I feel that it could be suggested that Foucault was gazing into the mirror when he made these observations.

A particular view of reason

Foucault is satisfied with a very careful empirical investigation of any discourse in the context of the practical field in which it is mobilised and in terms of the transformations it might bring about (see earlier discussion). All of this is very important. However, I find it too restrictive and too potentially pessimistic. I do not share Foucault's apparent fear that all reason and therefore all knowledge must always and everywhere be contaminated with a will to power, though I do not deny for a moment that it can be, may be, and often is; and that furthermore a careful empirical analysis can show this. However, unlike Foucault, I am not influenced by Nietzsche and his critique of reason, of which Foucault himself says,

> Examining the history of reason, he learns that it was born in an altogether 'reasonable' fashion...devotion to truth and the precision of scientific methods arise from the passion of scholars, their reciprocal hatred, their fanatical and unending discussions, and their spirit of competition – the personal conflict that slowly forged the weapons of reason. Further, genealogical analysis shows that the concept of liberty is an 'invention of the ruling class', and not fundamental to man's nature or at the root of his attachment to being and truth.
>
> (1980: 78)

There are a number of things to be said about this. First and foremost is the simple fact that if this is what one thought about reason then one would abandon it. It would then be 'reasonable', since reason was always and everywhere a product of competition, fanaticism and personal conflict, to be keen, but nevertheless content, to uncover that fact wherever possible. Reason produces discourse, reason is contaminated so therefore must discourse be contaminated and it is to this fact that the philosopher/historian/archaeologist in his/her work tries to draw attention. If on the other hand one had more faith in reason, then there would be more to be said. For instance, it might be that the discourse that one encounters does not suffer from *too much* reason – that is, fanaticism, will to power, rivalry etc. – but *too little* reason, that is, not enough truth, not enough rigour of method, or it may be insufficiently just etc.

There is an obvious sense in which these two views are incompatible, that is, if the two are set up in binary opposition. If we place *all* our faith in reason we will never see in discourse any of what Foucault or Nietzsche before him saw. If on the other hand we have no faith at all in reason we bar ourselves from asking further questions – there is only power and the will to truth. The question then becomes: do we have to choose one view or the other? We do not – there are other views, but before elaborating them it is necessary also to make some observations about the Nietzschean position, which informs the work of Foucault.

It is true that philosophers cannot be held responsible for the use to which their ideas are put, and it would be quite wrong to imply otherwise. For all of that, what follows is critical of the position on account of the inescapable fact of the Holocaust. In Auschwitz there was no reason, there was no justice and there was no truth, or if there was, then the Nazis wanted to murder it along with the countless thousands of people they murdered there. The truth that Auschwitz was an extermination camp remained as

> 348,820 suits of men's clothes,
> 836,525 women's dresses,
> 5,255 pairs of women's shoes,
> 38,000 pairs of men's shoes,
> together with great quantities of tooth brushes, shaving brushes, articles of everyday use, artificial limbs, spectacles, etc.
>
> (Smolen 1982: 39)

It is hard to begin to grasp its horror for those incarcerated and murdered in this place without reason, without truth, and without justice and it was these things that it lacked; this place was beyond reason. It is because of this that reason should not be abandoned, or justice and truth along with it. Perhaps when we are faced with an abundance of reason, rationality, knowledge and, often its unwelcome underside, power/knowledge, we can forget what life might be like without it, or its ultimate 'court of appeal'.

Though a philosopher cannot be held responsible for the use to which his ideas are put it is nevertheless also true that people who are no doubt less able, nevertheless have a responsibility to at least recognise the danger and alert others to it.

THE UTILITY OF THE CONCEPT OF IDEOLOGY

The Frankfurt school – a different view of reason

This is not to say, that reason is always and everywhere innocent. It is not. It may be too 'instrumental', as the Frankfurt theorists suggest, that is, unreasonable in its highly rationalised goal-seeking activity. Perhaps Horkheimer and Adorno (1972; first edition 1944) put the matter clearly when they suggest that

> The dilemma that faced us in our work proved to be the first phenomenon for investigation: the self destruction of the Enlightenment. We are wholly convinced – and therein lies our petitio principii – that social freedom is inseparable from enlightened thought. Nevertheless, we believe we have just as clearly recognised that the notion of this very way of thinking, no less than the historic forms – the social institutions – with which it is interwoven, already contain the seed of the reversal universally apparent today. If enlightenment does not accommodate reflection on this recidivist element then it seals its own fate. If consideration of the destructive aspect of progress is left to its enemies, blindly pragmatized thought loses its transcending quality, and its relation to truth.
>
> (p. xiii)

This seems to me to be a great advance upon the position taken by Nietzsche; however, it also seems both too pessimistic and too optimistic at the same time. The writers are, given the period, in understandable yet unhelpful despair; for instance, they suggest that in the

> culture industry the individual is an illusion not merely because of the standardisation of the means of production. He is tolerated only so long as his complete identification with the generality is unquestioned. Pseudo-individuality is rife; from the standardized jazz improvisation to [etc.]... what is individual is no more than the generality's power to stamp the accidental detail so firmly that it is accepted as such.
>
> (p. 154)

There is no agency here, the audience are passive victims. The commodity form of mass entertainment has overtaken them completely. Hence it is also too pessimistic. More than that, it seems that it is in the end false. But within all of this pessimism there is yet a massive optimism, because while it is said that 'self preservation in the shape of class has kept everyone at the stage of species being' (p. 155), a reader is nevertheless told, appropriately enough, in the very last sentence of Chapter 1, that the problem can be solved when 'Enlightenment which is in possession of itself and coming to power can break the bounds of enlightenment' (p. 208).

This is, it seems to me, the Hegelian Transcendental Subject. Here it is Enlightenment, pure thought, reason and true knowledge. In Lucaks it is all of these things embodied in the proletariat – perhaps it is here too – but not explicitly. Critical *theory* could not be called critical Marxism or it would risk its place in the academy. Either way the problem of German philosophy is elegantly resolved, at least on paper, in Chapter 1 by Spirit, or Reason, or the Proletariat, or all three since they are in this context identical in their function.

It is, in essence, this that Althusser (1971) criticised when he suggested

> What thus seems to take place outside ideology (to be precise, in the street), in reality takes place in ideology. What really takes place in ideology seems therefore to take place outside it. That is those who are in ideology believe themselves to be outside it; one of the effects of ideology is the practical denegation of the ideological character of ideology by ideology. Ideology never says; 'I am ideological'.
>
> (p. 175)

or when he suggests earlier that '1. There is no practice except by and in ideology. 2. There is no ideology except by the subject and for subjects' (p. 170).

The above can be grasped in two ways. At one level it could be seen as the same sort of pessimistic collapse that is involved in the idea of 'the masses' being the passive victims of the 'culture industry' – only now they are the hapless dupes of ideology. On the other hand it can be seen sensibly as a reproach to the idea of a transcendental subject which can suddenly see with pristine clarity all historical confusion, and serves as a (teleological) guarantee of progress in the end. There is no such guarantee. It is not the case that history is a carpet with a guarantee of progress woven into its pile. Neither is it the case that progress is forever ruled out by the iron grip of ideology.

As has been suggested earlier, it is important not to confuse the transcendental subject of history with the individual living breathing subject, that is, a person. It is hard to believe in a singular subject of history which becomes conscious of itself and of all history hitherto, that is, becomes a historical embodiment of pure reason etc. Nevertheless this emphatically does not mean that *individual subjects*, either as individuals or collectives, cannot become conscious of their social predicament and base their practice on better reason. Perhaps all people, not just an elite, can transcend previous ideological thought and base their practice on something much better, more real but, perhaps, there are no people, not even an elite, who can jump out of their skins and avoid all ideological consciousness at all times, always and forever, since, people are not gods.

Applying the Foucauldian theory of power/knowledge

Any attempt to apply the most pessimistic version of power/knowledge would involve attempting to establish that the originators or bearers/modifiers of a particular discourse were simply motivated out of a will to power in the Nietzschean sense, that is, 'devotion to truth and the precision of scientific methods arise from the passion of scholars, their reciprocal hatred, their fanatical and unending discussions, and their spirit of competition' (Foucault 1980: 78). In the context of the discourses considered in the following chapters this judgement would simply be far too harsh. This does not mean that discourse analysis itself need be rejected. However, it is important at this point to further elaborate the objections to a too literal version of power/ knowledge.

On page 49, there is a brief extract from the text of the guidebook through the museum of Auschwitz. It is a deeply sad text, since it describes in detail the horrors which took place inside Auschwitz. It is also a sad text because it is in an important sense a Stalinist text. The text has references to the bravery of the German Communist Party, and no doubt that there were many brave people in its ranks, and also outside its ranks. On the other hand it has nothing to say about the Communist Party of the Soviet Union (CPSU) and the Hitler/Stalin pact. Perhaps soon this book will be rewritten. It serves now, however, to remind a reader of the *twin* dangers of Fascism and Stalinism. Foucault is similarly afraid when he says what he says earlier about the risk of 'totalisation', and this should be respected.

It has been suggested earlier that there exists a particular responsibility to be alert to dangers such as these. This need not mean, however, that it is too risky to think of 'society as a whole'. In fact it may be both necessary and desirable to think of society as a whole. Totalisation is not the same as totalitarianism. Frederic Jameson – a Hegelian Marxist – in addressing a conference put it like this: 'the French nouveaux philosophers said it most succinctly, without realizing that they were reproducing or reinventing the hoariest American ideological slogans of the cold war; totalizing thought is totalitarian thought' (Jameson 1988: 354). He later adds that

> The conception of capital is admittedly a totalizing or systemic conception; no one has ever met or seen the thing itself, it is either the result of a scientific reduction (and it should be obvious that

scientific thinking always reduces the multiplicity of the real to a small scale model) or the mark of an imaginary and ideological vision. But let us be serious; anyone who believes that the profit motive and the logic of capital accumulation are not the fundamental laws of this world, who believes that these do not set absolute barriers and limits to social changes undertaken in it – is living in an alternative universe; or, to put it more politely, is doomed to social democracy, with its now abundantly documented treadmill of failures and capitulations. Because if capitalism does not exist then socialism does not exist either. I am far from suggesting that no politics at all is possible in this new post Marxian Nietzschean world of micro politics – that is obviously untrue. But I do want to argue that without a conception of the social totality (and the possibility of transforming a whole social system) no properly socialist politics is possible.

(Jameson 1988: 354–5)

While there is no reason to be scornful of micro-politics, certainly not if that involves helping to facilitate the counter discourse of the victims of local power, it nevertheless seems irresponsible to leave the matter there. The current war in Iraq, for instance, is not local. It is not total, but it might well have been. It was certainly total for the population of Baghdad, which remains a capital city with very little left in the way of an infrastructure. To be involved only in a local politics of the kind that Foucault envisages, important as such practice in itself is, would be at an important level to fiddle while Rome burned, or worse, it would be to surrender the globe to the forces that seem to be destroying it. This is a good reason for remaining committed to the concept of a social totality and to a critical Marxism which attempts to explain it.

This means, in the context of this book, investigating the utility of the concept of *both* discourse analysis *and* ideology in relation to the discourses contributing to, and contained within, the particular Acts of Parliament that are the subject of the book. Hence the book owes a debt to a critical appreciation of both Foucault and Marx. Nevertheless, as Hall (1988: 68–9) suggests,

I want to undermine the notion that theory consists of fully clarified concepts that are in a box in somebody's attic and one day you go up and open Pandora's Box and let the truth out. I want to suggest that theorizing is a process – the operation of scientific concepts on the ground of theoretical ideologies – that always operates by deconstructing existing paradigms and at the same time snatching important insights from what it is tossing out. So it has a necessarily mixed nature. You recover things that stand in the wrong place in the old conceptual matrix but that nevertheless give you insights into aspects of society and culture you did not have before. You have to reposition them.

The application of the concept of ideology

It remains important, however, to specify the way in which the concept of ideology will be used. It will be used, alongside discourse analysis, as a different and additional level of criticism of the discourses under consideration in the book.

Larrain (1979) reminds us of the importance of remembering that merely because ruling ideas may be in some important sense ideas of the ruling class, 'this does not make all of them ideological' (p. 50). Hence a procedure would be required for the ideological analysis of 'ruling ideas'. One procedure for the ideological analysis of such ideas, whatever they concern, would be to illustrate the ways in which such ideas, in order to give anything like an accurate account, need to grasp the (real) relations of production, and to show how the particular theory would be transformed if it was informed by this fact. In the process the way in which such ideas currently are of benefit to the ruling class would also need to be specified.

However, this is only clear when and where the focus is upon issues which bear a direct relationship to the relations of production which Marx set out to analyse. It is less clear when it comes to forms of domination which may not have a direct relationship to the means of production, for example, gender and sexuality. Indeed it is this perceived absence which has in part produced the outgrowth of work upon the question of ideology.

This absence is an important one in itself. It is also important because much of the discourse under consideration in this book takes familialism and the position of women and daughters within it as very much a taken-for-granted reality. Hence classical Marxism, though it is not as reductionist as it sometimes appears to be in the radical social-work literature, or as hopelessly deterministic as Rojek *et al.* (1988) imply that it is, nevertheless is not in itself fully adequate to the task of analysing all of the discourse under consideration in this book.

Hence, the concept of ideology which is used in the following chapters is not the classical Marxist concept. Rather it is indebted to the

Frankfurt school of Marxism, and it arises out of a desire, while maintaining a Foucauldian commitment to attending to empirical detail and to considering discourse which has power implications for individuals as individuals, nevertheless to resist what seems to me to be the Nietzschean excess of rejecting reason altogether. In other words it is not sufficient simply to uncover the potential effects upon individual subjects of the particular reasoning within the discourses under consideration, though that is important. There are also other ways to engage in critique, because

> Although we may wish to endorse the view that Foucault's conception and analysis of power–knowledge is not equivalent or reducible to the conception which has informed the work of the critical theorists, namely of a relationship between knowledge and ideology, this in no way exhausts the grounds of comparison between the respective positions.
>
> (Smart 1983: 135)

Smart continues by suggesting that

> The concept of critique has at least two different meanings in the work of the critical theorists, and whilst one of these undoubtedly signifies a process of reflection on humanly produced illusions, distortions, and systems of constraint – what might be described as a critique of ideology – another deeper sense, derived from the Enlightenment, is present in critical theory, namely of 'critique as oppositional theory as an activity of unveiling or debunking' ... It is this latter sense which I believe is implied in Foucault's reference to his work as a form of critique.
>
> (p. 135)

There are two points to be made about the above. Taking the latter conception of critique first, for all the seeming similarity to the position of Foucault it nevertheless remains clear that there is involved in it a commitment to reason. It is permissible in using it to argue that not only does the discourse imply this or that potential power effect, but *also* that it may be faulty in that it may contain insufficient reason and not simply an excess of it.

Taking into consideration the stronger conception outlined earlier, that is, that of a critique of ideology, it should be noted that there is the additional implication that, intentionally or unintentionally, a particular discourse may be true or false, but *in addition* it may, intentionally or unintentionally, serve the interests of the powerful over the less power-ful. This view of the matter maintains a more optimistic view of reason than that which is embodied in the Nietzschean tradition. It is also more optimistic on a political level in the sense that it is not afraid of thinking of a totality. As has been suggested earlier, while I am not scornful in the least of micro-politics, I nevertheless have a strong desire to avoid slid-ing into the idea that these are the only politics possible, since in my view to do so would risk a slide into a postmodernist excess that leaves the macro-political field entirely unoccupied by opposition. In addition I am far from sure that the rejection of macro-politics is not symptomatic of a pessimism born out of the political defeats of recent years (see Callinicos 1989: 162–74 and Eagleton 1991: 205).

Systematically distorted communication

The notion of systematically distorted communication as developed by Jurgen Habermas has a potential utility in developing a critical under-standing of the discourse under consideration because he draws attention to the possibility of an entire discursive system being warped out of true by the impact of the material world outside of discourse. For Habermas discourse is interactive and entering it means that one is prepared, outside all ulterior motive and constraint, to attempt an agreement. On this basis genuine discourse depends upon a rational consensus the attainment of which is, for Habermas, possible. It is also possible to recognise a true consensus and differentiate it from a false one, and it is only via such rational consensus that truth claims can be evaluated. All of this is only possible, however, where there is freedom from constraint or domination. This in turn means that *truth itself*, as he formulates the concept, can only be established where we are free from domination, and it is this freedom from domination that constitutes the 'ideal speech situation'. This serves as the standard via which systematically distorted communication can be measured. It is the case for instance in all of the discourse that is analysed in this book that the subjects/objects of the discourse do not have the right to speak – and this would have implications for the nature of the commu-nications that constitute the discourse, and therefore for its 'truth' claims.

However, there is an objection to this view. It is quite simply that it would be hard to imagine a situation in which all participants in a dis-course could be truly equal participants, and hence free from domina-tion. It is not the case that all conflict, and power differences between, for instance, men and women or adults and children, can simply be seen as a result of systematically distorted communication at a societal level. This is because 'the identification of power as a medium of exchange between the state-administration and the lifeworld obscures power relationships within the lifeworld itself' (Ashenden 1990: 19).

This is important in the context of the discourses under consideration in this book. The fact that there are power differentials *within* families and households may not be explained or even apparently recognised by a theory which appears to assume that in the absence of systematically distorted communication all will be well.

A further criticism of this position is that it is very close, if not identical, to the Hegelian transcendental subject. It is as if a whole society can overcome all the obstacles to rational communicative action. The transcendental subject is in this case all the members of a particular society who are suddenly guided only by reason. The same objections can be levelled against this position as can be levelled against the Hegelian transcendental subject, that is, it contains a far too optimistic view of pure reason.

Critical language study

The work of Fairclough (1989) is more helpful in this context since it offers a version of discourse analysis which he terms 'critical language study' which mobilises the work of, among others, Antonio Gramsci, and hence retains a commitment to a concept of ideology. For Fairclough ideology

> is most effective when its workings are least visible. If one becomes aware that a particular aspect of common sense is sustaining power relations at one's own expense, it ceases to be common sense, and may cease to have the capacity to sustain power inequalities, i.e. to function ideologically. And invisibility is achieved when ideologies are brought to discourse not as explicit elements of the text, but as the background assumptions which on the one hand lead the text producer to 'textualise' the world in a particular way, and on the other hand lead the interpreter to interpret the text in a particular way. Texts do not typically spout ideology. They so position the interpreter through their cues that she brings ideologies to the interpretation of texts – and reproduces them in the process.
>
> (Fairclough 1989: 85)

It is certainly the case that in much of the discourse under consideration in this book there exist unexamined common-sense assumptions about the role of families, and these certainly reinforce the existing power relations within families and households. However, the discourse under consideration does not construct or *constitute* these power relations within families and households. It is rather that in *taking them for granted* it *reinforces them*. In other words the power differentials in question already exist prior to the discourse. As Fairclough suggests earlier, the readers are situated in such a way by the text that they might well have a propensity to share the background common-sense assumptions contained within it. This is not the same as the discourse's itself constituting these assumptions. This seems to be a case very much akin to the one outlined earlier by Fairclough, and hence the additional use of the concept of ideology as well as that of power/knowledge is of utility in analysing the discourse under consideration.

With the addition of this concept of ideology to discourse analysis it becomes possible to suggest that a bearer of a particular discourse may bring to that discourse particular common-sense assumptions that lead the bearer of the discourse to bear that discourse uncritically. Hence it deepens the critique by enabling a dual focus: a focus on the discourse itself and, in addition, a focus on the bearer of the discourse. Eagleton (1991) suggests that

> Ideology is a matter of 'discourse' rather than of 'language' – of certain discursive effects. It represents the point where power impacts upon certain utterances and inscribes itself tacitly within them . . . a concept of ideology aims to disclose something of the relation between an utterance and its material conditions of possibility.
>
> (p. 223)

Another avenue of exploration is the work of Freud

> Freud has little to say directly of ideology; but it is very probable that what he points to as the fundamental mechanism of the psychical life are the structural devices of ideology as well. Projection, displacement, sublimation, condensation, repression, idealization, substitution, rationalization, disavowal; all these are at work in the text of ideology, as much as in dream and fantasy; and this is one of the richest legacies Freud has bequeathed to the critique of ideological consciousness.
>
> (Eagleton 1991: 185)

It may well be the case that any one or several of these mechanisms may be in play in the text of any given discourse.

In summary the discourse analysis in the following pages will be eclectic in the sense that it will follow the procedure for theorising that Hall (1988) quoted earlier offers. It will nevertheless owe a debt to both Foucault and Marx in that it will utilise elements of the concept of discourse analysis and of ideology, as defined earlier. In particular it will resist a total mistrust of all reason, and it will endeavour in every possible way not to lose sight of human agency, while nevertheless giving power its theoretical due in recognising the way in which it is productive of discourse that both subjectifies and objectifies. It will attempt above all to provide a more nuanced account of the development of British childcare legislation than is available in the existing social-work texts which are reviewed earlier and considered throughout the book.

This uncovering of a more detailed account owes a considerable debt to discourse analysis, since it is only by close scrutiny and analysis of the discourse itself that such an account is rendered possible. The book clarifies the central importance throughout 70 years of British childcare legislation of the struggle of the discourse of treatment over that of punishment. However, it also looks beyond the discourse itself since it attempts to outline the consequences of this for social work, social workers and the subjects/objects of their intervention. This aspect of the book owes a debt to the Frankfurt school of Marxism since it criticises the reasoning involved in the discourse without abandoning belief in reason itself. This is necessary because the discourses involved in British childcare legislation are of a consistently instrumental nature, and in order better to see this and the attendant consequence less instrumental reason is required.

The book also clarifies the centrality of familialism within British childcare legislation, and here a debt is owed to the concept of ideology as variously theorised and criticised earlier. This is because the notion of familialism is not *invented* by the authors and bearers of the discourses under consideration; rather it is brought to the discourse by them. This has the effect of reinforcing familialism by enshrining it in legislation.

Chapter 3

Still walking the tightrope?

This chapter considers the tragic case of Victoria Climbié and the Public Inquiry that followed. Lord Laming chaired the Inquiry and the Report was published in January of 2003. The government responded by producing the Green Paper *Every Child Matters*, and this formed the basis of the Children Act 2004. The Green Paper and the new Act will also be considered, both in the context of the original argument of the book, and of course in its own terms. The chapter concludes that because Lord Laming sees the 1989 Children Act as essentially sound legislation this leaves the competing discourses contained within it, and the resultant conflicting duties of social workers, intact. Lord Laming focuses instead almost solely on the issue of the better implementation of the 1989 Children Act (often through the recommendation of new managerial measures in order to do so). This reinforces the relevance of the following chapter which considers that Act in detail. This chapter also argues that the Government has missed an opportunity to strengthen the voice and the rights of children and young people within the child-protection system by failing to implement the UN Convention on the Rights of the Child.

The Victoria Climbié Inquiry Report

In common with the Maria Colwell Report some 32 years previous to it, the Laming Report offers its readers a narrative. It is headed: *Victoria's Story*. It is important to outline the main trajectories of this deeply sad story. The following account focuses on the significant elements of the narrative contained in the Inquiry Report (Laming 2003: 17–31).

The narrative

Victoria Adjo Climbié was the fifth of seven children and was born near Abidjan in the Ivory Coast on 2 November 1991. By all accounts she was happy and well cared for during the first six years of her life. However, her father's aunt (Mrs Marie-Therese Kouao), who had lived in France for a period but was visiting the Ivory Coast for the funeral of her brother, told Mr and Mrs Climbié that she wished to take a child back to France with her and arrange for his or her education. Victoria was chosen, though another young girl called Anna was the first choice, but her parents changed their mind. Victoria was chosen instead and she was named as Anna and presented as a 'daughter' on the French passport used by Mrs Kouao.

In France, Victoria was enrolled at the Jean Moulin primary school in Villepinte. However her attendance soon became very irregular and, in 1999, a Child at Risk Emergency Notification was issued. A social worker assigned to the case suggested that the relationship between Victoria and Mrs Kouao was difficult.

In the spring of 1999, Mrs Kouao told the school that she was taking Victoria to London so that she could receive treatment for a dermato-logical condition. A forwarding address was given, and it was that of a Ms Ackah, who was a distant relative of Kouao's. Victoria went to say goodbye to her classmates on 25 March 1999, and the Head Teacher noticed that she was wearing a wig – her head had been shaven.

Victoria arrives in the UK

Kouao and Victoria boarded a flight from Paris to London on 24 April 1999. They travelled on Kouao's French passport, in which Victoria was described as her daughter. The picture in the passport was not that of Victoria but Anna, the child she had replaced. Perhaps Victoria's head was shaved and she was made to wear a wig so she looked more like the child in the passport photograph. There was no immigration record of their arrival because they travelled as EU citizens. They went to Acton and moved into a double room in a bed and breakfast hotel.

On 25 April 1999, Victoria and Kouao visited Ms Ackah. Victoria was introduced as 'Anna'. Ms Ackah noticed that Victoria was wearing a wig. Later that day on a visit to Victoria and Mrs Kouao, Ms Ackah's daughter, Ms Quansah, took the wig from Victoria's head. This revealed that she had no hair and that her scalp was covered with marks. Though both mother and daughter thought that Victoria looked small and frail, they did not notice anything to concern them about Victoria or her interaction with Mrs Kouao.

The following day, Kouao and Victoria went to Ealing's Homeless Persons' Unit. They needed somewhere to live when their initial reservation in the bed and breakfast ran out. They were accommodated in a hostel, into which they moved into in May 1999.

Over the next few weeks, Victoria and Kouao visited Ealing Social Services on a number of occasions in order to collect subsistence payments. Mrs Kouao often complained about their accommodation. In this period a number of staff who saw Kouao and Victoria noticed that Kouao was always well dressed whilst Victoria was anything but that. A person named Deborah Gaunt, who once saw them, went as far as to say that Victoria looked like an 'advertisement for Action Aid'.

Victoria did not attend school and as far as is known had no friends. On 8 June 1999 Kouao took Victoria to a doctor's surgery on Acton Lane, Harlesden. No physical examination of Victoria was undertaken because she was said not to have any health problems. It was felt that there were no child-protection concerns that required follow-up or reporting to other agencies.

Six weeks after first encountering Victoria, Ms Ackah, who had not seen Victoria since her visit, bumped into her and Kouao on the street on or around 14 June 1999. Victoria had only her face and hands exposed because of the long dress that she was wearing. There was a fresh scar on Victoria's right cheek. Kouao told her this had been caused when Victoria fell on an escalator.

Later that same day, Victoria met Carl Manning for the first time. According to Manning, he gave Kouao his telephone number after a conversation with her that took place on a bus that he was driving. She called him a few days later and invited him to visit her. Their relationship lasted until their arrest just over 8 months later.

In the meantime Ms Ackah was concerned by what she had seen of Victoria in the street, and also that her accommodation was unsuitable for a child. It was dirty and cramped. She was worried about Victoria's weight. A man who lived at the accommodation told Ms Ackah that he was concerned about the way Kouao treated Victoria. As a result of all of the above, Ms Ackah made the first anonymous telephone call, of two, to Brent Social Services.

Victoria and Mrs Cameron

By the middle of June, Victoria was being looked after in the daytime by Priscilla Cameron, who was an experienced but unregistered child minder. Kouao was working at the Northwick Park Hospital. Victoria would usually arrive at her childminder at around 7 am and be collected on occasions as late as 10 pm.

Victoria was treated well by Mrs Cameron. Her English improved and she apparently had a good relationship with Mrs Cameron's adult son, Patrick. Mrs Cameron had concerns about the way Victoria was treated. For example, Kouao would often speak very harshly to her. On one occasion, when Mrs Cameron mentioned to Kouao that Victoria would sometimes move things around in the house, when she should not, she was upset that Kouao shouted at Victoria that she was a 'wicked girl'. This attributing of 'wickedness' to Victoria was often repeated. Ultimately demonic possession was unhelpfully advanced as an explanation for Victoria's incontinence.

Mrs Cameron's concern was not diminished by a conversation she had with a woman she referred to as 'Nigerian Mary', who asked Mrs Cameron what it was that she had said to Mrs Kouao that gave her cause to beat Victoria every night. In addition, Victoria would become very quiet and reserved and anxious when Kouao arrived at the house to take her home. Mrs Cameron also noticed that Victoria often had a number of small cuts to her fingers. Kouao told Mrs Cameron that Victoria had been playing with razor blades. Mr Cameron also noticed marks to Victoria's face, although these were not serious and he thought they could have been caused by ordinary play.

Victoria moves into Carl Manning's flat

On 6 July 1999, Victoria and Kouao moved into Manning's flat. There was a separate bathroom and kitchen area, but only one room, and two sofa beds. Ominously, on 13 July 1999, Kouao asked Mrs Cameron to care for Victoria permanently because Manning did not want her living with him. Mrs Cameron declined, but she agreed to take Victoria for one night because 'the poor child was looking so ill'. Mrs Cameron was given two large bags full of Victoria's clothes.

On arrival, Victoria had a cap pulled down over her face. Mrs Cameron removed it and she saw what she thought was a burn on Victoria's face. Mr Cameron noticed three marks on Victoria's jaw that looked to him 'like injuries that had been healing for a little while'. Victoria's eyes were bloodshot, and there was a loose piece of skin hanging from her right eyelid. Mrs Cameron's asked Kouao who had burned and beaten the child, and she replied that all the injuries were self-inflicted. Manning, however, later told the police that Victoria began to suffer from urinary incontinence soon after she came to live in his flat. He told the police that this is why he hit Victoria. He recalled that he began by slapping her, but by the end of July he had started using his fist.

Later that evening, Mrs Cameron heard groaning coming from the room in which Victoria was sleeping. Victoria was asleep, but her face was swollen and her fingers were oozing pus. Mrs Cameron, the next morning, took Victoria to see Marie Cader, a French teacher at her sons' school, in order to seek advice about the injuries. Victoria was reluctant to talk about them. It was decided that Victoria needed hospital treatment.

Victoria's first visit to hospital

On 14 July, at Central Middlesex Hospital, Victoria was seen by a Dr Beynon. Dr Beynon took a history from Ms Cameron and undertook a basic examination of Victoria. He was concerned and he referred Victoria to a paediatric registrar. The paediatric registrar who saw Victoria was Dr Ekundayo Ajayi-Obe. She discovered a large number of injuries to Victoria's body, which she recorded on a set of body maps. Dr Ajayi-Obe arranged for Victoria to be admitted overnight and called Brent Social Services to inform them. Victoria was placed under police protection at 5.20 pm. Unsupervised visits by Victoria's mother (Mrs Kouao) were forbidden.

When Mrs Kouao discovered from the Camerons that Victoria had been admitted to the Central Middlesex Hospital, she went to the hospital and was there when Dr Ruby Schwartz saw Victoria. Dr Schwartz diagnosed Victoria as suffering from scabies. Victoria was nursed in isolation for the rest of her stay.

The next morning, after the police protection had ceased, Kouao took Victoria away from hospital. Subsequently they went to the Camerons' house to collect Victoria's clothes. Victoria did not respond to being spoken to by either of the Camerons and she seemed 'totally different' from other times that Mr Cameron had seen her. Apart from one occasion when Mrs Cameron saw Kouao and Victoria walking together down the street, this was the last time that the Camerons' saw either of them again.

Victoria's second visit to hospital

On 24 July 1999, Victoria was admitted to the North Middlesex Hospital. She had a serious scald to the face. Kouao said that the scald was caused by Victoria trying to relieve the itching caused by scabies by placing her head under a hot tap. Victoria's burns were so serious she was admitted to the paediatric ward – known as Rainbow ward – where she stayed for 13 nights. At about 11 pm on 24 July 1999, Dr Simone Forlee, the senior house officer who first examined her, explained the position to Haringey Social Services. A more detailed referral was made 3 days later by Karen Johns, an Enfield social worker based at the hospital. As a result, a strategy meeting was held at Haringey's offices on 28 July 1999 and Victoria's case was allocated to a social worker.

A number of medical staff who were caring for Victoria during her stay on Rainbow ward noticed marks on her body which they considered were signs of serious deliberate physical harm. This was also indicated by her behaviour in the presence of Kouao and Manning. The relationship between Victoria and Kouao was recorded in the ward's critical incident log as being like that of 'master and servant'. On one occasion she was seen to wet herself while standing to attention in front of a seated Kouao, who was telling her off. Her reaction to Manning when he came to visit appears to have been much the same.

Ms Arthurworrey (Victoria's social worker) and PC Karen Jones visited on 6 August 1999 and they spoke briefly to Victoria and decided it would be appropriate for her to be discharged back into Kouao's care. She left the North Middlesex Hospital with Kouao on that day. They went back to Manning's flat in Somerset Gardens where Victoria was to spend the remaining 7 months of her life.

The social worker's first home visit

Victoria's had little or no contact with anybody other than Manning and Kouao, and professionals saw her on only four times in her last 7 months. The first two times were home visits made by Ms Arthurworrey. The other two occasions were at the beginning of November when Kouao took Victoria to Haringey Social Services where she alleged that Victoria had been sexually abused by Manning. She later withdrew the allegation.

The first of Ms Arthurworrey's two visits to the flat took place on 16 August 1999. Though she did not talk to Victoria during the visit, she formed the impression that Victoria was happy. She felt that her priority was to move Kouao and Victoria to alternative accommodation.

Mr and Mrs Kimbidima

Some time in July, Kouao met a man on the street, both spoke French, and the man, Julien Kimbidima, invited Kouao back to his house to meet his wife, Chantal. Kouao visited the Kimbidimas on 2 August 1999 and, shortly after Victoria's discharge from hospital, Kouao took her to meet

Mr and Mrs Kimbidima. Victoria was quiet and withdrawn, and she started to cry when Kouao told Mrs Kimbidima that Victoria was not her real daughter. The Kimbidimas saw Victoria a number of times over the following months, and Mrs Kimbidima sometimes looked after Victoria. When at the Kimbidimas' house, Victoria would sit quietly in the corner, as she was told to do so by Kouao. Once or twice she wet herself while at their house. Mrs Kouao would shout at Victoria, show no warmth or affection, and she told Mrs Kimbidimas that Victoria was 'possessed by an evil spirit'.

Victoria, the church and her exile to the bathroom

On 29 August 1999, Kouao and Victoria attended the Mission Ensemble pour Christ, where the pastor was Pascal Orome. He had a detailed rec-ollection of Victoria's appearance at this stage. Victoria was dressed in heavy clothing that covered all of her body apart from her head and hands. The pastor advised Kouao to cut Victoria's hair shorter so that the injuries that he had noticed to her scalp could 'breathe'. Kouao told him about Victoria's incontinence. He thought she was possessed by an evil spirit, and suggested prayer as a remedy. When she told him a fortnight later that the problem, after a brief improvement, remained, he appar-ently reproached her for being insufficiently vigilant and allowing the evil spirit to return.

It was at that time that the sofa bed Victoria had been sleeping on was thrown out and she was forced to sleep in the bathroom. The bathroom was small and there was no window and no heating. The bathroom door was kept closed and the light was off. Victoria spent her nights alone, in the cold and dark.

The second social work visit

At his trial, Carl Manning described the second visit of Ms Arthurworrey as 'a put up job'. The flat had been made clean and tidy in preparation for the prearranged visit. The social worker neither saw nor smelt any evidence of Victoria's incontinence. Manning said that Victoria was told how to behave in front of the social worker. The pair said that Victoria was sleeping on the remaining sofa bed, with Manning and Kouao sharing a new bed on the other side of the room.

At the end of the visit, Victoria suddenly jumped up and shouted at Ms Arthurworrey. She said words to the effect that she (Ms Arthurworrey) did not respect her or her mother, and that they should be given a house. This behaviour surprised Ms Arthurworrey at the time. During the course of their conversation, Ms Arthurworrey told Kouao that the council only accommodated children who were 'at risk of serious harm' and that, in the council's view, Victoria was not at such risk.

The sexual abuse allegation

Three days later, Kouao contacted Ms Arthurworrey to make allegations that Manning had been sexually abusing Victoria. At the social worker's office, Kouao cited three instances of sexual abuse. Victoria, when spoken to alone, repeated the allegations almost word for word. So much so that Ms Arthurworrey and the other social worker present, Valerie Robertson, thought she had been coached. Lisa Arthurworrey said that Victoria did not seem to be 'a particularly nervous, frightened or fearful child' at this meeting.

Mrs Kimbidima was contacted in an endeavour to arrange for Victoria to be cared for elsewhere during the investigation. Victoria and Kouao left the office in a taxi to the Kimbidimas' house. However, by the end of the day they had returned to Somerset Gardens. They withdrew their allegations the following day. Kouao was told that, despite the retraction, she and Victoria would have to live elsewhere during the investigation. Kouao said that she and Victoria could continue to stay with the Kimbidimas. Instead they returned to their own flat. This was the last time any of the professionals involved in Victoria's case saw her before her admission to hospital on the night before her death.

Victoria's last four months

Apart from two trips to France, it would seem that Victoria spent most of this 4-month period in the Somerset Gardens flat. Victoria continued to be forced to sleep in the bath and, from November onwards, she was, by all accounts, 'tied up' inside a black plastic sack, apparently to stop her from soiling the bath. On New Year's Eve, an entry in Manning's diary describes an argument with Kouao which ended by her returning to his flat in order to 'release Satan from her bag'. Poor Victoria obviously had to lie in her own urine and faeces for long periods. In a police interview, Manning said that he was worried that the state of Victoria's skin might cause social workers to ask 'undue questions'. This may have led to the abandonment of the plastic bag, though apparently in his evidence to the Inquiry he couldn't remember why the change was made.

Nevertheless, Victoria began to spend more and more of her time in the bathroom, she continued to sleep in the bath, but she also spent some of her days in it as well. Kouao and Manning began to serve Victoria her meals in the bath, her hands were bound and hence, she was forced to eat like a dog.

Victoria was also beaten on a regular basis, using a variety of implements, including a shoe, a hammer, a coat hanger and a wooden spoon. The police found traces of Victoria's blood on the walls, on Manning's football boots and on one of his trainers. He apparently also used a bicycle chain. In early 2000, Victoria's parents received a Christmas card from Kouao in which were photographs of a smiling Victoria, and they were told that 'She's growing up well and she finds herself... well'.

Victoria returns to church

A pastor from north-west London, Pat Mensah, recalled that Victoria seemed 'a bit poorly' when she visited Somerset Gardens on 12 February. Ms Mensah indicated that she was concerned about Victoria's health and advised that she be taken to hospital. She also advised that Victoria should be taken to a church and on 19 February 2000 Kouao took Victoria to the Universal Church of the Kingdom of God housed in the old Rainbow Theatre on Seven Sisters Road. When they arrived they were shouting at each other and Victoria appeared to find it hard to walk. They were disturbing the service, so Victoria was taken to the crèche. Victoria was shivering and when asked if she was cold, Victoria replied that she was hungry. Victoria was given some biscuits. She hid them in her pocket.

At the end of the service, Pastor Lima spoke to Kouao about Victoria's incontinence. Again, it was said that an evil spirit possessed Victoria. Kouao was advised to bring her back to church on the following Friday because this was the day on which prayers are said for deliverance from 'witchcraft, bad luck and everything bad or evil'.

On the next Sunday, Kouao and Victoria returned to the church where a Pastor Celso Junior saw them. Apparently, Victoria was quiet during the visit. On the following Wednesday, Kouao phoned Pastor Lima and told him Victoria's behaviour had improved in that she had ceased to cover the flat in excrement. On Thursday, Kouao phoned the church and said that Victoria had been asleep for two days and had not eaten or drunk anything. By the evening of that day, Kouao brought Victoria to the church and asked for help. Pastor Lima advised them to go to the hospital and a minicab was called.

Victoria's final visit to hospital

Mr Salman Pinarbasi, the minicab driver, was so worried about Victoria that he took her straight to the Tottenham Ambulance Station. She was delivered by ambulance to the casualty unit of the North Middlesex Hospital. She was unconscious and very cold. Her temperature was dangerously low.

A Dr Lesley Alsford was called in to take responsibility for Victoria's treatment. Her examination of Victoria was limited because her first wish was to increase Victoria's temperature, which at this point was 28.7 degrees Celsius. Victoria needed intensive-care facilities of the sort unavailable at the North Middlesex. Victoria was transferred to St Mary's Hospital, Paddington. She was in a critical condition with severe hypothermia and multi-system failure. Her respiratory, cardiac and renal systems began to fail. Cardio-pulmonary resuscitation was attempted but all endeavours to save her failed. She was declared dead at 3.15 pm on 25 February 2000. She was 8 years and 3 months old.

The post-mortem examination

A post-mortem examination was carried out on the following day. The cause of death was hypothermia, which had been caused by malnourishment, a damp environment and restricted movement. There were 128 separate injuries on Victoria's body. There were marks on her wrists and ankles that showed that her arms and legs had been tied together. It was the worst case of deliberate harm to a child the doctor had ever seen.

The arrest

Kouao was arrested on suspicion of neglect at the hospital around 11.35 pm on 25 February 2000. She told the police, 'It is terrible, I have just lost my child'. Carl Manning was arrested the following afternoon as he returned to his flat. Both were later charged with Victoria's murder and were convicted at the Central Criminal Court on 12 January 2001. They are currently serving sentences of life imprisonment.

Lord Laming's response

Reading Lord Laming's response to the above narrative a reader is struck by his barely concealed anger and indignation. In the Introduction to the

Report under the heading *What Went Wrong?* Lord Laming has this to say:

> I recognise that those who take on the work of protecting children at risk of deliberate harm face a tough and challenging task. Staff doing this work, need a combination of professional skills and personal qualities, not least of which are persistence and courage. Adults who deliberately exploit the vulnerability of children can behave in devious and menacing ways. They will often go to great lengths to hide their activities from those concerned for the well-being of a child.
>
> (Laming 2003: p. 3)

He adds that staff often

> have to cope with the unpredictable behaviour of people in the parental role. A child can appear safe one minute and be injured the next.
>
> (p. 3)

However, he then points out that

> Whenever a child is deliberately injured or killed, there is inevitably great concern in case some important tell-tale sign has been missed.
>
> (p. 3)

He nevertheless maintains that

> Those who sit in judgement often do so with the great benefit of hindsight. So I readily acknowledge that staff who undertake the work of protecting children and supporting families on behalf of us all deserve both our understanding and our support.
>
> (p. 3)

After this display of understanding for the dilemma that social-work and social-welfare professionals face, Lord Laming nevertheless distinguishes that case of Victoria from all others. He describes it as 'altogether different' and he finds it 'deeply disturbing' that in the period following her first contact with Ealing Housing Department's Homeless Persons' Unit

> Victoria was known to no less than two further housing authorities, four social services departments, two child protection teams of the Metropolitan Police Service, a specialist centre managed by the

NSPCC, and she was admitted to two different hospitals because of suspected deliberate harm.

(p. 3)

He considers that the 'dreadful reality' was that these agencies knew very little more about Victoria at the end of this process than they did when she was first referred. He considers that

> The final irony was that Haringey Social Services formally closed Victoria's case on the very day she died.

(p. 3)

Lord Laming considers that the failure to protect Victoria was 'lamentable' and suggests that her protection 'required nothing more than basic good practice being put into operation' (p. 4). A reader is then informed that Neil Garnham QC listed 12 occasions when the relevant services had the opportunity to intervene positively on behalf of Victoria, and furthermore many other opportunities came to light during the enquiry and that none of these required 'great skill' or would have made significant demands on time (p. 4).

Lord Laming tells us that what took place was 'a gross failure of the system' in which none of the agencies involved emerge with 'much credit', because 'they gave a low priority to the task of protecting children'. Whilst he recognises that the agencies involved were 'underfunded, inadequately staffed and poorly led', he nevertheless tells the reader that he remains

> amazed that nobody in any of the key agencies had the presence of mind to follow what are relatively straightforward procedures on how to respond to a child about whom there is concern of deliberate harm.

(p. 4)

A reader is informed that the Deputy Assistant Commissioner of the Metropolitan Police Service, William Griffiths was highly critical of the investigation carried out by Haringey (police) Child Protection Team, saying that 'In the A to Z of an investigation, that investigation did not get to B' (p. 4). This leads Lord Laming to observe that in spite of the Children Act 1989 having been in force for almost 10 years, the investigation into criminal offences against children 'may not be as rigorous as the investigation of similar crimes against adults' (Laming 2003: 4).

Under the heading, 'Widespread Organisational Malaise', the report moves to consider the performance of the medical professionals. Whilst accepting that paediatric doctors and nurses are very well trained in helping sick children and that child abuse is one of the most complex areas of paediatrics and child health Lord Laming adds,

> That being so, I found it hard to understand why established good medical practice, that would have undoubtedly helped clarify the complexities in Victoria's case, was not followed on the paediatric wards at the Central Middlesex Hospital and North Middlesex Hospital.
>
> (pp. 4–5)

Management issues

In considering management issues, Lord Laming commences by apportioning differential levels of criticism between the 'handful of hapless, if sometimes inexperienced, front-line staff', whose work was 'generally of very poor quality', and the 'managers and senior members of the authorities' to whom he directs, 'most criticism'. He suggests that

> It is significant that while a number of junior staff in Haringey Social Services were suspended and faced disciplinary action after Victoria's death, some of their most senior officers were being appointed to other, presumably better paid, jobs. This is not an example of managerial accountability that impresses me much.
>
> (p. 5)

He later adds that

> The most lasting tribute to the memory of Victoria would be if her suffering and death resulted in an improvement in the quality of the management and leadership in these key services.
>
> (p. 6)

Under the heading *Moving Forward* Lord Laming points out that his brief went beyond the merely 'forensic' analysis of what went wrong. The Inquiry had also been charged with looking forward and making recommendations for 'how such an event may, as far as possible, be avoided in the future' (p. 7).

Managerialism and the Victoria Climbié Inquiry Report

In considering the recommendations of the report, and the Government's response to them, it is important to recognise that Lord Laming does not criticise the 1989 Children Act. Indeed, in his speech introducing his report on 28 January 2003 he explicitly informed his audience of that fact – 'I have concluded that the current legislative framework is fundamentally sound. I am persuaded that the gap is in its implementation'.

He adds, 'I am in no doubt that that this Inquiry Report must have as its primary objective that it will bring about a major change in the way that these key public services are managed'.

Whilst an improvement in management is in itself be something to be welcomed, nevertheless, an exclusive and isolated focus on this issue can be characterised as managerialism. Managerialism (Clarke *et al.* 2000; Muncie and Hughes 2002; Parton 2004) is characterised by an emphasis on developing connected, coherent and effective sets of policies and practices, often rhetorically referred to as 'joined up services'. Cost-effectiveness is also centrally important in managerialism. It is governed by pragmatism and not by any particular philosophy. This enables complex moral and philosophical issues to be sidestepped in favour of a pragmatic 'what works' approach. It involves both a high level of centralism and a simultaneous devolution, the setting of targets, the development of performance indicators and the putting in place of core competences against which the performance of agencies and their staff are measured. There is also an emphasis on strong leadership. It is an ethos in which multi-agency cooperation, and risk-assessment strategies are welded together in an all embracing 'task-centred environment' which focuses on audit, performance targets, cost-effectiveness, accountability and evidence-based practice.

As Lord Laming in his speech put it:

> Those in senior positions carried, on behalf of us all, the responsibility for the quality, efficiency and effectiveness of the service delivered. They must be accountable for what has happened. That is why their posts exist.

It is clear that his focus is very much on managerial issues. These can of course be helpful, but not at the expense of a deeper analysis. The problem with the managerialist response is not at all what such a response may encompass; it is rather that it risks overlooking important wider, and potentially more deep-seated, problems. In this specific case, it fails to critically examine the competing ideologies and discourse contained in the 1989 Children Act, instead focusing on an improved implementation of it. This is best illustrated by further considering Lord Laming's Report, and some of the key recommendations.

Three basic propositions

The Laming Report made 108 recommendations, and in his speech to Parliament he summarised them. He informed Parliament that 'more exhortation that services should work better together is not enough', adding that 'in order to achieve the level of change I consider to be necessary I advance three basic propositions'.

The first proposition calls for fundamental change 'in the capacity of the management of each of these key public services'. The second proposition calls for a clear and unambiguous line of managerial accountability from top to bottom.

The third proposition is that the current Area Child Protection Committees should be replaced, and there should be a new National Agency for children and families with powers to ensure that all of the key services carry out their duties in an efficient and effective way.

The achievement of the above three proposition require some 'radical change'. Some of the key recommendations are outlined immediately later.

A Children and Families Board

With the support of the Prime Minister, a ministerial Children and Families Board should be established at the heart of government. The Board should be chaired by a minister of Cabinet rank and should have ministerial representation from government departments concerned with the welfare of children and families.

A National Agency for Children and Families

The chief executive of a newly established National Agency for Children and Families will report to the ministerial Children and Families Board. The post of chief executive should incorporate the responsibilities of the post of a Children's Commissioner for England.

The newly established National Agency for Children and Families should have the following responsibilities:

- to assess, and advise the ministerial Children and Families Board about, the impact on children and families of proposed changes in policy;
- to scrutinise new legislation and guidance issued for this purpose;
- to advise on the implementation of the UN Convention on the Rights of the Child;
- to ensure that legislation and policy are implemented at a local level and are monitored through its regional office network;
- to report annually to Parliament on the quality and effectiveness of services to children and families, in particular on the safety of children.

At a local level – committees for children and families

Each local authority with social-services responsibilities must establish a Committee of Members for Children and Families with lay members drawn from the management committees of each of the key services. This Committee must ensure the services to children and families are properly coordinated and that the inter-agency dimension of this work is being managed effectively.

A Management Board for Services to Children and Families

The local authority chief executive should chair a Management Board for Services to Children and Families which will report to the Member Committee referred to above. The Management Board for Services to Children and Families must include senior officers from each of the key agencies. The Management Board must also establish strong links with community-based organisations that make significant contributions to local services for children and families. The Board must ensure staff working in the key agencies are appropriately trained and are able to demonstrate competence in their respective tasks. It will be responsible for the work currently undertaken by the Area Child Protection Committee.

The Management Board for Services to Children and Families must appoint a director responsible for ensuring that inter-agency arrangements are appropriate and effective and for advising the Management Board for Services to Children and Families on the development of services to meet local need. Furthermore, each Management Board for Services to Children and Families should establish reliable ways of assessing the needs and circumstances of children in their area, with particular reference to the needs of children who may be at risk of deliberate harm.

The unexamined discourses

In concluding that the 1989 Act is 'basically sound legislation', Lord Laming therefore focuses on developing a child-protection system that more efficiently administers and operates that legislation. In this sense, his response is essentially managerialist and it leaves intact the 1989 Act in all of its essentials. The competing discourses of punishment and prevention still exist in tension with each other and become integrated into the duties of social workers. The tensions between support for families, and prevention of child abuse, and the surveillance of families, and the detection of child abuse, remain unchanged. Of course it would be greatly to be welcomed if these tensions were better managed, and if front-line workers were to receive much better support and management. Nevertheless, it is hard to imagine that a situation in which social workers intervene, to either too little an extent or too great an extent, will be eliminated. This is especially true if the competing discourses remain unexamined and unacknowledged.

Competing and contradictory discourses – the UN Convention on the Rights of the Child

It is sometimes tempting for academics to overstate the coherence and unity of their objects of study and this risks missing the contradictions and nuances involved in them. On the other hand, there are good grounds not to treat ideologies and discourses simply as random sets of ideas, or equally random pieces of knowledge. This is important in the context of the Laming Report and subsequent legislation that is based upon it, because there is in the report, alongside its central managerialist thrust, another very important discourse. The recommendation that a Children's Commissioner be appointed, one of whose duties is to advise on the implementation of the UN Convention on the Rights of the Child, brings into play a discourse of human rights and in particular children's rights. This is most certainly to be warmly welcomed because it may be that a very strong statutory focus on the rights of children and young people could do much to reduce their maltreatment at the hands of adults, whether those adults are their parents or even governments, who may maltreat children by illegal invasions of their home countries. It is necessary therefore to consider the Government's response to Lord Laming and consider it in this context.

The government's response to Lord Laming's report

The government response to Lord Laming's report, entitled *Keeping Children Safe*, was published together with a Green Paper entitled *Every Child Matters*, in September of 2003 (Department of Health 2003: Cm 5860). Green Papers are consultation documents, and they are followed by White Papers, which are statements of intended legislation, which in turn become Bills, which are placed before Parliament. When the Bill is passed it becomes an Act of Parliament. The Children Act 2004 brought into law the Government's responses to the Laming report, which were in essence contained in the above Green Paper.

Every child matters

The Green Paper offers an Executive Summary. Under the heading *Past Failings,* a reader is told that the death of Victoria Climbié exposed 'shameful failings in our ability to protect the most vulnerable children'. Furthermore it becomes instantly clear to a reader that the government shares Lord Laming's managerialist approach, because we are told that

> From past inquiries into the deaths of Maria Colwell and Jasmine Beckford to recent cases such as Lauren Wright and Ainlee Walker, there are striking similarities which show some of the problems are of long standing. The common threads, which led in each case to a failure to intervene early enough were poor co-ordination, a failure to share information, the absence of anyone with a strong sense of accountability, and frontline workers trying to cope with staff vacancies, poor management and a lack of effective training.
>
> (p. 5)

A wider and more ambitious reach – a new discourse of prevention?

Because 'as Lord Laming's recommendations make clear', the issue of child protection, 'cannot be separated from policies to improve children's lives as a whole', the Green Paper goes on to outline policies not only to protect children but also to 'maximise their potential'. A framework is set out for children and young people from birth to the age of 19 who live in England. A reader is informed that the proposals 'aim to reduce the numbers of children who experience educational failure, engage in offending or anti-social behaviour, suffer from ill health, or become teenage parents'. Hence the need to protect children at risk is set 'within a framework of universal services which support every child to develop their full potential and which aim to prevent negative outcomes' (p. 5).

> The Government inform readers of the Green Paper that young people, children and families had been consulted, and:
> The five outcomes that mattered most to children and young people were:
> **Being healthy**: enjoying good physical and mental health and living a healthy lifestyle. **Staying safe**: being protected from harm and neglect. **Enjoying and achieving**: getting the most out of life and developing the skills for adulthood. **Making a positive contribution**: being involved with the community and society and not engaging in anti-social or offending behaviour. **Economic well-being**: not being prevented by economic disadvantage from achieving their full potential in life.
>
> (pp. 5–6)

These outcomes are pursued in the Green Paper by acting on four main areas and they are: *Supporting Parents and Carers, Early Intervention and Effective Protection, Accountability and Integration – locally, regionally and nationally and Workforce Reform.* The proposals under each of these headings are summarised below.

Supporting parents and carers

This is to be accomplished through 'universal services', that is, schools, health services and childcare:

> providing information and advice and engaging parents in supporting their child's development, where such support is needed or wanted. In addition there are envisaged 'targeted and specialist support to parents of children requiring additional support', and 'compulsory action through Parenting Orders as a last resort where parents are condoning a child's anti-social behaviour such as truanting or offending'.
>
> (p. 39)

Early intervention and effective protection

The Green Paper points out that Victoria Climbié came to the attention of a number of agencies, and that none of them 'acted on the warning signs'. Hence it seeks to improve the sharing of information between agencies by developing a database so that that all local authorities have a list of children in their area, and a list of any services that they have had contact with, together with the contact details of relevant professionals (p. 51).

A 'common assessment framework' is promised within which 'core information' will 'follow the child between services to reduce duplication'. A 'Lead professional' will be identified in order to coordinate in cases where a child is 'known to more than specialist agency'. Multidisciplinary teams will be formed in which the professionals responsible for identifying children at risk will be integrated, and services will be 'co-located "around" schools, Sure Start Children's centres, and primary care settings'. Effective child-protection procedures will put in place 'across all organisations' (p. 51).

Together these measures are intended to raise the 'priority of safeguarding children amongst all relevant organisations' (p. 64). It should be noted that safeguarding is a wider remit than that of protection. It has a strong preventative focus and it is proactive. It requires that all agencies working with children take all reasonable steps to ensure that risks to the welfare of a child is minimised. In addition there would be an obligation in cases where concerns about such risk is identified for all agencies to take action to address those concerns, and all working in partnership to the agreed policies and procedures. Whilst this endeavour is to be welcomed it is nevertheless appropriate to signal that, as in all overarching preventative endeavours, it may at crucial times be a tall order and like all tall orders it is at least possible that it, at times, may not be met.

Accountability and integration – locally, regionally and nationally

The aim here is that a single person should be identified, locally and nationally with the responsibility 'for improving children's lives'. This will be accomplished by the creation of a Director of Children's Services, accountable for local authority education and children's social services. In addition 'a lead council member for children' will be put in place. In the longer term 'Children's Trusts' will be created, which under a Director of Children's Services will integrate local authority education, children's social services, some children's health services, and other appropriate agencies and services, for example, Youth Offending Teams. These will be part of the local authority and will report to elected members. The local authorities will be expected to work closely with private and voluntary agencies in order to 'improve outcomes for children' (p. 67).

In addition to the above 'Local Safeguarding Children's Boards' will replace the current Area Child Protection Committees. These developments will be supported by a Minister for Children Young People and Families in the Department for Education and Skills. A new duty to safeguard children and promote the well-being of children will be given to 'local bodies such as the police and health organisations' and local authorities will be given a duty to promote the educational achievement of children in care (p. 68).

The intention is stated to set out 'clear practice standards expected of each agency in relation to children'. An Integrated Inspection Framework for Children's Services, led by Ofsted, will be created. These joint inspection teams will 'ensure that services are judged on how well they work together'. It is envisaged that 'performance will be driven up by sharing effective practice and intervening where services are failing' (p. 68).

The children's commissioner

A reader is informed that real service improvement is only attainable through involving children and young people and listening to their views (p. 68). In pursuit of such an outcome a Children's Commissioner who will act as a 'children's champion' is advocated. The Commissioner 'would speak for all children, but especially the disadvantaged whose voice is too often drowned out' (p. 79).

Another function of the Commissioner is to involve children and young people in developing services. This is seen as a way to create 'an organisation defined by its client group rather than professional functions' and produce 'bottom up pressure for change' (p. 78).

Whilst bottom-up pressure for change and an organisation defined by its client group, are to be warmly welcomed, it also needs to be recognised that the overall proposals in the Green Paper do not amount to producing either of these things. Indeed, the proposals overall reflect the strong centralised managerialism of the recommendations of Lord Laming. Furthermore the proposals for the Children's Commissioner fall significantly short of Lord Laming's recommendation on the subject since there is no mention of the role of the Commissioner to advise on the implementation of the UN Convention on the Rights of the Child. This is a significant step backward from empowering children and young people to have a meaningful voice and real rights, not only within child-protection and youth-justice policy, but also throughout the wider society itself. This makes the Green Paper's claims concerning bottom-up pressure for change or an organisation defined by its client group, ring rather hollow.

Workforce reform

Under this heading, the Green Paper advocates a 'workforce reform strategy' the purpose of which will be to increase the effectiveness, skills, training, retention and recruitment of the 'children's workforce'. In order to accomplish this

> A Children's Workforce Unit, based in the Department for Education and Skills, will develop the pay and workforce strategy for those who work with children. The Unit will work with the relevant employers, staff and Government departments to establish a Sector Skills Council (SSC) for Children and Young People's services to deliver key parts of the strategy.
>
> (p. 83)

No one could reasonably object to better training and a better career structure aimed at recruiting and retaining the social workers who face the daunting task of supporting children and their families whilst simultaneously policing and detecting child abuse, especially given the tragic consequences which all too often happen, and which form the central focus of this book. Having freely acknowledged this, it is important to recognise that the proposals in the Green Paper follow the managerialist approach of Lord Laming. The Green Paper therefore suffers from the same potential fault line of the Laming Report in that it leaves the ideologies and discourses within the 1989 Children Act unexamined and intact. Thus, the critical examination of that piece of legislation, which is the subject of Chapter 4 of this book, remains highly relevant. The remaining work of this chapter is to consider the way in which the Green paper's proposals were brought into legislation.

The 2004 Children Act

The Act gained Royal Assent on 15 November 2004. The overall aim of the Act is to produce greater accountability for children's services, to enable improved efficiency in joint working and to create a stronger emphasis on the safeguarding of children. Part 1 of the Act establishes and defines the role of the Children's Commissioner. Part 2 of the Act brings into law the proposals set out in the Green Paper considered earlier, designed to bring about more integrated and better-planned services for children. Part 3 and 4 of the Act introduces similar provisions to Part 2, relating specifically to Wales whilst reflecting the different more devolved context. Part 5 deals with miscellaneous provision, including strengthening the current notification arrangements for private fostering. The Act will be briefly commented upon under all of its relevant sections.

Part I Children's Commissioner

Section 2 of Part 1 of the Act concerns the functions of the Children's Commissioner, and the primary function is to promote awareness of the views and interests of children in England.

Furthermore, the Commissioner, in considering the for the purpose of her/his function under s2, what constitutes the rights and interests of children – '. . . must have regard to the United Nations Convention on the Rights of the Child (s. 2(11))' (Smith 2005: 9).

Whilst this is an improvement on the proposals in the initial Green Paper, it is nevertheless important to remember that having regard for a Convention is not the same as advising upon the implementation of it, which was what Lord Laming recommended – or, most important of all, resourcing it. The implementation of the Convention would have very far-reaching and positive implications for children and young people and it is therefore appropriate here to consider the background to this issue.

The UN Convention on the Rights of the Child

This Convention has been ratified by 192 states – only the US and Somalia has not done so. It contains 54 Articles of which 40 give direct rights to children, and the remainder concern measures of implementation. It was adopted by the UN General Assembly in 1989, and the UK ratified the Convention, with all party support, in 1991. In the same year, the Committee on the Rights of the Child, which is an international body of 18 children's rights experts elected by the State Parties, published guidelines for the preparation of progress reports on implementation by State Parties. In 1995 and 2002, the Committee on the Rights of the Child provided a comprehensive report on the UK's progress in implementing the Convention. The report in 2002 *(Committee of the Rights of the Child – Consideration of the Reports Submitted by States Parties Under Article 44 of the Convention – concluding observations: United Kingdom of Great Britain and Northern Ireland (CRC/15/Add.188))* was overall very critical and made no less than 78 recommendations, which the UK government would need to implement, in order to make their policy and practice compatible with the Convention.

The Children's Rights Alliance of England, a highly respected federation of more than 230 voluntary and statutory children's rights organisations, produces an annual review of the UK government's action in relation to the earlier report. It is appropriate to consider some aspects of their review of 2005, particularly those that relate to the 2004 Children Act.

In the 2005 review, whilst welcoming the appointment of Professor Al Ainsley-Green as England's Commissioner they nevertheless have this to say:

> England's new Children's Commissioner has the weakest general functions in the UK and Europe – promoting awareness of children's views and interests, rather than promoting and safeguarding their rights.
>
> (p. 18)

In addition to the above, the Commissioner is the least independent in the UK; for instance the Secretary of State can direct the Commissioner to carry out an inquiry. On the other hand, the Commissioner must consult the Secretary of Sate if he wishes hold an independent inquiry. None of the above is the case for the Commissioner in Wales, Northern Ireland or Scotland.

The Committee on the Rights of the Child in their 2002 *Concluding Observations* called upon the UK Government to 'Incorporate into domestic law the rights principles and provisions of the Convention' (p. 3). However in the 2004 Children Act the UK government focused, instead of this, on the five broad outcomes goals outlined in *Every Child Matters*. Had they instead focused upon a plan of action on the implementation of the Convention they would have potentially produced far stronger child-protection measures. For instance Article 12 of the Convention says,

1   *States Parties shall assure to the child who is capable of forming his or her own views the right to express those views freely*

in all matters affecting the child, the views of the child being given due weight in accordance with the age and maturity of the child.

2 *For this purpose, the child shall in particular be provided the opportunity to be heard in any judicial and administrative proceedings affecting the child, either directly, or through a representative or an appropriate body, in a manner consistent with the procedural rules of national law.*

Clearly this places an obligation on all concerned with direct work with children to consult with them on all matters that impact upon them. This centralises the rights of the child within child protection, and indeed on all other matters of relevance to their lives. It is surely worth remembering, in relation to the tragic story of Victoria Climbié, that Victoria was known to three housing authorities, four social services departments, two child-protection teams of the Metropolitan Police Service, a specialist centre managed by the National Society for the Prevention of Cruelty to Children (NSPCC) and two different hospitals, because of suspected deliberate harm, and that these services apparently knew little or nothing more about Victoria at the end of the process than at the beginning of it. Tragically, Haringey Social Services Department closed Victoria's case on the day she died.

A social-work practice that was driven by the human rights of Victoria, under the UN Convention, in particular article 12, might have avoided this tragic outcome, if only for the simple reason that it would require a direct one to one engagement with the child, by all who came into professional contact with her. Sadly, it would appear that this level of engagement was missing in this distressing case, and this, independently of any particular organisational arrangements, might have saved her life.

It may be objected that there can exist a genuine conflict between the rights of adults and the rights of children. However, in relation to this, it should be remembered that the Human Rights Act of 1998 places an obligation on all courts in England and Wales to, as far as is possible, interpret all legislation, whenever enacted, in a way which is compatible with the European Convention on Human Rights. In other words it would be unlawful for public authorities to act in a way that is incompatible with Convention rights. In relation to child protection, article 8 of the above Convention is often raised, frequently on the behalf of parents, but also in some cases in relation to children, which concerns the Right to Respect for Private and Family life. Whilst tension between the rights of adults and children can at times exist, there is an obligation in legal proceedings to respect all human rights. This would not be diminished by the implementation of UN Convention of the Rights of the Child. The UN Convention has been critiqued (see for example, Freeman 1993), as being a compromise, as too dependent on individualistic Western conceptions of rights, and as lacking any teeth with which to enforce it, giving it a semblance of a grand but ineffective gesture. However it does provide a tool to enable policy makers and lobbyists to put pressure on governments, and a benchmark against which to measure progress. Furthermore, whilst formal legal rights are not always a guarantee that such rights can be 'cashed', their existence can nevertheless be an important 'lever' which might well assist in doing so, and is far better than a situation where such formal legal rights do not exist at all.

Part 2 children's services in England

Part 2 of the Act brings into law the main proposals contained in *Every Child Matters*. As outlined in the consideration of the Green Paper above, it introduces a duty on local authorities to make arrangements through which key agencies cooperate in order to improve the well-being of children and places a responsibility upon those agencies to have regard to the need to safeguard children and promote their welfare. It introduces statutory 'Local Safeguarding Children's Boards' to replace the non-statutory Areca Child Protection Committees. The power to create a national database that will contain basic information on all children is introduced. A requirement is placed upon English local authorities that they put in place a Director of Children's Services who will, at the minimum be responsible for education and social services in so far as they relate to children, and also a lead council member for children's services, who will have political responsibility for these services within the local elected council. An integrated inspection framework for children's services, making possible joint area reviews of all services in a given area (Smith 2005: 2), is also created.

All of the above closely follows the recommendations of Lord Laming. As has been observed above, the proposals are essentially managerial in their approach. The almost exclusive focus on managerialism is in the end an insufficient response to the tragedy which, like so many childcare tragedies prior to it, provoked the need to legislate. It represents a missed opportunity to strengthen the rights of all children and young people by implementing the UN Convention of the Rights of the Child, and developing social-work practice, policy and the development of services, in this context.

Only time will tell whether these new arrangements will offer better and more integrated services for children and young people. It is important to remember that this is not the first time that centralisation has been a response to tragedy. The Curtis Committee, appointed in 1945 was influential in the production of the 1948 Children Act (see Chapter 5 of this book). This Committee recommended the setting up of a new committee at the time within the local authority, called the Children's Committee. This, it said, would give 'additional strength to the recommendation that a Children's Officer of similar status to a Medical Officer of Health be appointed to each Children's Committee' (p. 46). Clearly, the centralisation of children's services in itself does not guarantee improved outcomes for children because this depends on the quality of the delivery of service by the professionals involved. And this, whilst it can be improved by particular organisational and managerial arrangements, cannot be guaranteed by those arrangements, whatever form they may take. In relation to this issue, the programme of workforce reform, designed to produce better training, and enhanced status for the children's workforce is of course to be warmly welcomed, since it should produce better service delivered to children and their families. What is also required is the kind of overall macro-social and economic change for children and young people, and enhancement of their status, that the implementation of the UN Convention would bring about.

Part 5 of the Act introduces miscellaneous provisions. One of these provisions (s. 53) is explicitly concerned with extending the extent to which children and young people are consulted about their wishes and feelings in relation to services provided to them under s.17 of Children Act 1989. Clearly this is a step forward, though of course if article 12 of the UN Convention on the Rights of the Child were in force, that obligation would be greatly reinforced since it would apply to all children and young people.

A children's rights-based social-work practice requires a view of children and young people not only as vulnerable and in need of protections, which of course they all too frequently are, but also, alongside that, a view of children and young people as citizens (Neale 2004), like all other citizens, who, with proper regard to their age, understanding and best interests, have the same human rights as the rest of us. The societal view of childhood has changed frequently throughout history (Hendrick 2003). This seeing the child as also a citizen requires different channels of recognition and respect in which there is a need to reach an authentic understanding of the other – in this case, children and young people (Assiter 2003: 95). This requires principles of recognition and respect in welfare provision (Williams 2000: 352, 358) that recognise, listen to and makes every endeavour to act upon the voice of the recipient of services, in this case children and young people. Whilst small incremental aspects of this position are present within the legislation and discourse considered above, sadly, they play a 'bit-part' within the overall strategy and this is the lost opportunity and Achilles' heel of the discourse under consideration.

Chapter 4

The 1989 Children Act

A significant shift?

The current chapter considers some of the discourse arising out of a public enquiry, that is, the *Report of the Inquiry into Child Abuse in Cleveland 1987* (HMSO 1987a) as well as some of the discourse contained in the White Paper entitled *The Law on Child Care and Family Services* (HMSO 1987b). In addition, where necessary, it will also make reference to, and quote from, *Working Together – a guide to arrangements for inter-agency co-operation for the protection of children from abuse* (Department of Health 1991).

These documents remain of significance today, nearly 20 years after they were produced because of their importance in constructing what has been a dominant discourse, if not the dominant discourse, during the whole of that period and in many ways continues to be so, the 2004 Children Act notwithstanding, though a later edition of *Working Together* (Department of Health 1999) is briefly considered in Chapter 8.

This chapter focuses on these documents for a number of reasons. In the first place the events in Cleveland can be seen as significant in contributing to a legislative redrawing of the boundary between the State and 'the family', in the 1989 Children Act (see, for instance, Frost and Stein 1989: 75; Parton 1991: 151–2; Vernon 1990: 47).

It is also true that the events taking place in Cleveland from January to July of 1987 can be seen as a stark contrast to previous child abuse 'scandals'. In Cleveland, social workers and their agencies and manager, and members of the medical profession, were criticised for being over-zealous, and in the case of, for instance, Maria Colwell and many subsequent cases involving the tragic deaths of children, it was alleged that they were being insufficiently vigilant.

The White Paper referred to earlier requires specific consideration because it is an important official discourse in this apparent redrawing of boundaries. The official report into events in Cleveland was published later than the White Paper and it called for the urgent implementation of some of the recommendations of the *Review of Child Care Law* which reported in 1985, and upon which the White Paper was based.

Working Together – a guide to arrangements for inter-agency co-operation for the protection of children from abuse (Department of Health 1991) requires consideration because it calls for inter-agency cooperation in relation to matters of child abuse, both physical and sexual, and hence there may be a sense in which as a result social workers may not be quite as centralised in issues of child abuse as previously, though it remains the case that the 1989 Children Act lays upon social services departments a central duty to 'safeguard and promote the welfare of children "in need" and, so far as is consistent with that duty, to promote their upbringing by their families by providing a range and level of services appropriate to their needs' (see HMSO Children Act 1989 s.17).

REPORT OF THE INQUIRY INTO CHILD ABUSE IN CLEVELAND

The full report about the perceived crisis in Cleveland covers a total of 320 pages. This chapter considers the short version (Cleveland County Council 1988) extracted from the complete text. The short version does outline the narrative and the recommendations and conclusions in full, though it does not include a report of all of the evidence given by people appearing before the inquiry.

The narrative

The introduction to the Report itself points out that the inquiry arose 'from an unprecedented rise in the diagnosis of child sexual abuse in the months of May and June 1987 in the County of Cleveland, principally at Middlesbrough General Hospital' (p. 1).

It is clear from the report that there had been some tension between the police and other agencies involved in child abuse, which stretched back as far as 1985 and 1986. The Area Review Committee (a coordinating group with representatives of the various agencies involved in dealing with child abuse) was unable to gain agreement from the police for a new set of procedural guidelines (p. 2).

The Report also points out that Cleveland County Council Social Services Department appointed a Child Abuse Consultant, a

Mrs Richardson, in 1986 in order to 'give child protection a greater priority'. Dr Marietta Higgs was appointed soon afterwards as a consultant paediatrician in South Tees Health District. Prior to her arrival she consulted Mrs Richardson about the level of services available for 'deprived and abused children' (p. 2). She also contacted the Director of Social Services (Mr Bishop) and his Senior Assistant Director. She became the vice-chair of the Joint Child Abuse Committee which took over from the Area Review Committee.

In her previous post in Newcastle-upon-Tyne, Dr Higgs had examined two children who were in the care of Cleveland County Council, and she saw, what was for her the first time, 'reflex relaxation and anal dilatation'. A consultant paediatrician, Dr Wynne, had informed her that this was a sign which was found in children who had been sexually abused. On the basis of this sign, together with 'various physical findings', Dr Higgs diagnosed anal abuse (p. 2).

In South Tees, soon after her arrival, Mrs Richardson was consulted about a 6-year-old girl with vaginal bleeding. She first advised that a police surgeon be involved, but upon realising that the referring doctor was also a police surgeon, she referred the matter to Dr Higgs. Dr Higgs diagnosed sexual abuse, and the girl 'indicated that her grandfather was responsible' (p. 2). The grandfather, who was arrested and given bail conditional upon residence in a bail hostel, nevertheless denied the abuse.

One month later the girl was referred again with the same symptoms and the same diagnosis was made. At this point it is appropriate to quote the Report directly.

> The grandfather on this occasion could not be the perpetrator, and the little girl said it was her father. The police were embarrassed by this revelation and dropped the charges against the grandfather. Inspector Whitfield consulted the senior police surgeon, Dr Irvine. The police wanted to examine the child. Dr Irvine telephoned Dr Higgs. He said she refused to let him examine the child: He expressed the firm view that the signs were unreliable. On the following day both Dr Higgs and Dr Irvine were at the case conference. Dr Irvine again said he could not accept the grounds for the diagnosis and that Dr Higgs was placing too much reliance upon the observations of Drs Hobbs and Wynne.
>
> (p. 2)

Dr Irvine consulted a Dr Raine Roberts, who was a 'well known police surgeon from Manchester, she supported his stand' (p. 3).

The same girl was seen on two further occasions, each time the same symptoms were present, and on each occasion Dr Higgs took the view that they indicated further sexual abuse. On the fourth occasion the child was living with foster parents.

Anal dilatation

Later in that same month a boy of two was referred to the hospital by his family. He was suffering from constipation. Dr Higgs upon examining the boy found 'scars around the anus and the sign of anal dilation'. She therefore 'considered the possibility of sexual abuse' and asked the parents to bring in the elder brother and sister, aged 10 and 9 respectively, for examination. She found signs of anal abuse in the boy and vaginal and anal abuse in the girl. The Report points out that 'This was the first time that she had diagnosed sexual abuse on the basis of physical signs alone' (p. 3).

The children had not made a complaint of sexual abuse. Upon the request for a second opinion the children were examined by Dr Wynne in Leeds and she confirmed the diagnosis on the basis of the same signs that had led Dr Higgs to the same conclusion. The children had been photographed by a police photographer and 'the police later objected to the use of a police photographer for this purpose' (p. 3). After that, medical photographers were used.

The children were interviewed by the police. There was no social worker present at the interview. The eldest boy was at one point thought to be the 'possible perpetrator'. His father said the boy was 'grilled' by the police, and he was upset, and 'this was a matter of some concern to the social workers involved in the case' (p. 3).

The children were made subjects of a Place of Safety order and they were placed with separate foster parents. They were also made wards of court. An educational psychologist and social workers interviewed the children and they believed that the children made disclosures of sexual abuse by their father. However after the hearing they were returned to their family, since 'the Judge held that they had not been sexually abused' (p. 3).

The Report suggests that Dr Wyatt, a colleague of Dr Higgs who had little experience in child sexual abuse, was shown the sign by Dr Higgs, and 'he found it striking' (p. 3). In April Dr Wyatt himself diagnosed that a 3-year-old girl who had these signs was a victim of sexual abuse. This was the first occasion that he himself had observed the signs in one of his own patients. The Report continues to relate broadly similar stories of groups of children being referred and diagnosed as sexually abused in a similar manner. In May, for instance, 47 children were diagnosed as sexually abused. One father of three children was charged with 'several sexual offences and committed suicide while awaiting trial' (pp. 4–5).

All of this led to extreme pressure on both the hospital beds and foster placements and by June the Cleveland Social Services fostering officer 'became overwhelmed and ran out of space for the children'. The Hospital Unit Manager, Dr Drury, contacted both the Social Services Department and Dr Higgs in order to discuss the pressure on resources and the disagreement between Drs Irvine and Higgs. The Community Health Council expressed concern about 'public anxiety over the admissions to the hospital and the diagnosis of sexual abuse' (p. 5). Mrs Richardson, the Cleveland Social Service Department's Child Abuse Consultant, contacted the Director of Social Services and spoke of 'a crisis' (p. 5).

Mrs Richardson and members of the Social Services Directorate met to discuss the matter. However, Mrs Richardson did not report on the 'difference between Dr Higgs and Dr Irvine' (p. 5). The implication in the report is that this was important and should have been reported.

The final breakdown of relations between the police and the Social Services Department

The police, reinforced by the 'strong views of Dr Irvine', were in doubt about the diagnosis of sexual abuse and the anal dilatation test. Dr Irvine had made his view of the matter clear to the Chief Superintendent (p. 5). It should also be recollected that there was tension between Dr Higgs and the police photographers, who felt 'embarrassed' and also felt that the children were 'upset' (P. 5). There was a meeting between the Head of the Police Scientific Aids Department and Dr Higgs. However, it was 'more of a confrontation' (p. 5). There was also the view of the Police Community Relations Department, headed by Inspector Makepeace, that: 'the good relations which he believed existed between police officers and social workers on the ground had deteriorated since the appointment of Mrs Richardson in her new role' (p. 5).

At a further meeting of the Joint Child Abuse Committee (mentioned earlier), chaired by Mrs Richardson, the members of the committee were able to agree on most of the outstanding issues 'which had troubled their predecessors on the Area Review Committee' (p. 6). However, they were not able to agree on:

1   [T]he degree of co-operation between the police and social workers in the investigation of sexual abuse.

2   [W]ho should perform the medical examination and whether
    the police surgeon should be consulted.

(p. 6)

It was therefore agreed that Mrs Richardson and Chief Inspector Taylor
should convene a meeting at which both Dr Irvine and Dr Higgs would
be present, in order that some agreement may be reached. According to
the report this meeting did not go well. Dr Irvine had examined by now,
for the first time, some of the children who had been diagnosed as having been sexually abused by Dr Higgs. His findings were negative;
Dr Higgs on the other hand had had some confirmation of the diagnosis
from other paediatricians and she was 'convinced of the reliability of the
test' (p. 6). Dr Irvine expressed the view that 'Dr Higgs was incompe-
tent and misguided and that her "mentors" in Leeds, Dr Wynne and
Dr Hobbs, were equally misguided' (p. 6).

The Report then elaborates upon the consequences of this breakdown.
The police and the Social Services Department commenced to act
entirely independently of each other. After the meeting a memo was
drafted which was 'largely the work of Mrs Richardson'. It was sent to
the Director of Social Services who signed it. The consequence was to
'exclude the police surgeon from making a second examination', and
also to make provision for 'routine applications for Place of Safety
orders in cases of suspected sexual abuse', and to suspend parental
access in such cases (p. 6). The police on the other hand sent out a Force
circular instructing officers to view 'Dr Higgs' diagnosis on sexual
abuse with caution' (p. 6). Furthermore, 'neither agency informed the
other of the steps they were taking' (p. 6). In addition, the police representative on the Joint Child Abuse Committee was instructed by the
Assistant Chief Constable not to attend. The next meeting of that committee confirmed the exclusion of the police surgeon from examinations
in cases of suspected sexual abuse.

The Report indicates that in June 'children continued to be referred in
ever growing numbers, mainly by Social Services'. On 18 June there
was a confrontation at the hospital between 'an angry father' and
Dr Wyatt. A parents' support group was formed in that month, and Stuart
Bell MP became involved and visited the hospital on a number of
occasions.

By now, some of the Place of Safety orders were running out and
applications had to be made for interim Care Orders. This involved the
Magistrates Court. On one day in the Teesside court there had been
45 applications for interim Care Orders, many of which werebeing
contested, and in such cases the medical evidence being brought forward

was disputed. Concern was expressed by the magistrates (p. 8). Dr Higgs and Dr Wyatt were asked to 'hold back'. They refused on the grounds that if they 'saw child sexual abuse they had a duty to act' (p. 8). The two were interviewed on two occasions: once by three senior consultants and once by Professor Bernard Tomlinson, the chair of the Northern Region Health Authority, who could 'find no reason to recommend their suspension from duties' (p. 8). By now, at the request of Social Services, second opinions were being sought. Also the parents were seeking second opinions.

The matter was by 26 June a 'national issue'. Dr Irvine appeared on television and claimed Dr Higgs was 'wrong in her diagnosis of sexual abuse in respect of a particular family' (p. 9). Stuart Bell MP asked a question in the House of Commons on 29 June asking for a Ministerial statement on the 'recent increase in the number of cases of alleged child abuse in Cleveland' (p. 9). On 9 July the Secretary of State for Social Services ordered that a statutory Inquiry be established.

Conclusions and recommendations

Arising from the aforementioned narrative the Committee of Inquiry came to conclusions and made recommendations, and these will be outlined later, after which the links between these conclusions and the White Paper entitled *The Law on Child Care and Family Services* (HMSO 1987b) and the 1989 Children Act will also be outlined. It will then remain to consider the extent to which the Act may be thought to represent a significant shift in the boundaries between the 'family' and the law in British childcare legislation.

Part 3 of the Inquiry report is headed 'Final Conclusions', and in its first paragraph it informs a reader that

> We have learned during the Inquiry that sexual abuse occurs in children of all ages, including the very young, to boys as well as girls, in all classes of society and frequently within the privacy of the family...problem of child sexual abuse has been recognised to an increasing extent over the past few years.... This presents new and particularly difficult problems for the agencies concerned in child protection. In Cleveland an *honest attempt was made to address these problems* by the agencies. In Spring 1987 *it went wrong*.
>
> (p. 243, my emphasis)

In the paragraph immediately following the earlier one, the reasons for the crisis, which are seen as 'complex', are said 'in essence' to include

- a lack of proper understanding by the main agencies of each other's functions in relation to child sexual abuse;
- a lack of communication between the agencies;
- differences of views at middle management level, which were not recognised by senior staff. This eventually affected those working on the ground.

(p. 243)

Instrumental reason and the de-politicisation of sexual abuse

What should be immediately noticed about the earlier is the essentially instrumental, technical and managerial tone of the discourse. The problem of child sexual abuse is 'new' and therefore 'particularly difficult'. An 'honest' attempt was made to address these problems. However, 'it went wrong'. There is little here which points to the differential attitudes to the problem held by the police and hospital doctors. The issue is de-politicised by the discourse, and the solution advanced is an essentially technical/managerial one.

According to the report the central question is one of the main agencies' understanding each other's functions, of their communicating properly, and of managers' recognising differences of views and acting in good time. However, when one considers the narrative it could be concluded that the agencies were well aware of each other's functions, and they initially fulfilled those functions. Nevertheless, because of very different attitudes to the problem, they simply failed to agree, and thus failed to cooperate. The discourse reverses this process because it suggests that the failure to agree was a result of a lack of communication and cooperation between the agencies. In fact the failure to agree resulted in a breakdown of communication and cooperation.

Added to the above list of problems, that is, a lack of inter- and intra-agency cooperation, the Report criticises particular people. Dr Higgs is criticised because, after having made her initial diagnoses in the cases of the first few children, and after having had confirmation of these diagnoses from Dr Wynne: 'she proceeded with increasing confidence. The presence of the physical signs was elevated from grounds of "strong suspicion" to an unequivocal "diagnosis" of sexual abuse' (p. 243).

The Report adds that Dr Wyatt also became convinced of the reliability of the physical signs, and 'he enthusiastically supported her' (p. 243).

These two consultants thus became 'the centre point of recognition of the problem'. In all, 121 children from 57 families were diagnosed. The Report criticises the consultants in the following terms:

> By reaching a firm conclusion on the basis of physical signs and acting as they would for non-accidental injury or physical abuse; by separating children from their parents and admitting most of the children to hospital, they compromised the work of the social workers and the police. The medical diagnosis assumed a central and determining role in the management of the child and the family.
>
> (p. 243)

The Report suggests that the two doctors, while correctly playing their part in the identification of sexual abuse, nevertheless had a duty to examine their actions in order to consider whether those actions were in the 'best interests of the children and the patients' (p. 243).

However, it is of interest to contrast the conclusions of the Report to what the consultants themselves, writing in 1991, say.

> A doctor may make a medical diagnosis of sexual abuse on the basis of symptoms and signs. There may be no corroborative information and this may result in the case not going to court. Nevertheless the doctor should be able to say on the behalf of the child that there is a medical diagnosis of sexual abuse. In other cases, on the basis of symptoms and signs, the doctor may reach the opinion that sexual abuse is a differential diagnosis but that opinion will fall short of the degree of certainty required to make a medical diagnosis. In this way there would still be a flexibility for doctors to accurately express their opinion. If the multidisciplinary framework is strong it should be able to accommodate the full range of medical opinion. This would decrease the risk of scapegoating individual professionals when difficulties arise.
>
> (Wyatt and Higgs 1991: 36–7)

The two doctors quote Kerns (1989) on the question of the understandable pursuit of certainty on the behalf of agencies involved in this issue:

> Given the heated arena of adversary proceedings, media scrutiny, and passionate lobbies of all parties, it is not surprising that social

workers, police officers, lawyers, and judges have turned to medical examination in pursuit of 'certainty' in alleged child sexual abuse cases.

(Kerns 1989: 177)

The pursuit of certainty

The question the doctors raise is an important one. The Report criticises them for elevating a cause for strong suspicion into that of a certainty. However, is the pursuit of certainty simply their own? After all, the discourse of the Report suggests that they were correct in fulfilling their role, but had a duty to consider whether they were acting in the best interests of the child. However, it is hard to imagine that it would be always counter to the best interests of a child to make no diagnosis unless one was certain. On the other hand it would not be hard to imagine the trouble the doctors might have been in had they not made a diagnosis if it later transpired that a child was, in fact, being sexually abused. The subsequent management of the case, that is, the resolution of the question of what to do in the light of a particular diagnosis, is what raises the question of certainty.

The Report acknowledges that the two consultants were not responsible for the subsequent management of the cases and criticises the Cleveland Social Services Department Child Abuse Consultant, Mrs Richardson, who supported the consultants' approach. This is because she

Advised that immediately the diagnosis was made the child should be removed to 'a place of safety'.... This practice was confirmed by the issuing of a memorandum by the Director of Social Service which in practice had the effect of endorsing the medical diagnosis of the two paediatricians.

(pp. 243–4)

It should be noticed here that it is, in fact, the action of the removal of the children to a place of safety which had the effect of endorsing the medical diagnosis. In other words, the doctors were not their own judges. Hence the Report has the effect of shifting the responsibility for the pursuit of certainty from the Social Services Department to the doctors.

Differential standards of proof

It should be remembered that there is a differential standard of proof required in criminal proceedings as opposed to that required in care proceedings. The police, in order to secure a conviction, need a case which can be proved beyond reasonable doubt, which is much stronger than in the case of care proceedings, which are civil proceedings, and in which the standard of proof is less rigid, that is, on the balance of probability. Some of the tension between the Cleveland Police and the Cleveland Social Services Department can be accounted for by these differential standards of proof, though this is not to deny any potential role played by differential attitudes to the problem of child sexual abuse itself. It is also true that these differential standards of proof produce situations where a criminal prosecution for abuse is not achieved, even though it may go to trial, and nevertheless, later, a Care Order is granted. If the criterion of 'beyond reasonable doubt' was the only one available then some children could be left in abusive or potentially abusive situations.

It is not surprising either that the Cleveland Social Services Department looked to a medical diagnosis as producing hard evidence, particularly when it came from paediatricians who were known to have a strong commitment to dealing with the issue of child sexual abuse, since it is their responsibility to promote the welfare of the child and not primarily to secure a conviction. This is important because it arises out of a tension between the legislative imperative to secure a conviction, which arises out of the discourse of punishment, and a legislative duty to promote the welfare of children, which is much more related to the discourse of treatment. The fact that one may shade into its apparent other, for example, where a child may be removed from home in situations where there is not certainty of abuse, is not recognised by the Report. It is these complexities which the instrumental, technical and managerial tone of the Report masks.

Familialism and the discursive resolution of conflicting demands

The Report appears to recognise the difficulty of dealing with the issue of sexual abuse, and also appears to recognise the conflicting demands that are placed upon social workers. However, if it is to maintain its instrumental stance then the discourse must appear to resolve this conflict. It states that

> Those who have a responsibility to protect children at risk...have in the past been criticised for failure to act in sufficient time and to take adequate steps to protect children who are being damaged.

In Cleveland the general criticism of the public has been of overenthusiasm and zeal in the action taken. It is difficult for professionals to balance the conflicting interests and needs in the enormously important and delicate field of child sexual abuse.

(p. 244)

It also adds that

Social Services whilst putting the needs of children first must respect the needs of parents; they must also work if possible with the parents for the benefit of the children. These parents themselves are often in need of help. Inevitably a degree of conflict develops between these objectives.

(p. 244)

The language in play here is significant. We are told that children are being 'damaged', and that the 'field' of sexual abuse is 'enormously important'. However, it is also 'delicate'. Conflicting interests have therefore to be 'balanced'. Parents must be respected and worked with. We should notice here the genderless nature of the word parent. It is overwhelmingly men who sexually abuse and it is also the case that they may not be parents – they may be boyfriends of the child's mother, relatives, step-parents, etc. The discourse is situated within familialism – a familialism which suggests that in the enormously difficult and delicate area of sexual abuse the 'family' has to be worked with. There is a singular notion of a family in play in the discourse. Families appear to be places where the plural and genderless parents look after children. There is no recognition of the changing family/household form, or of the differential power and conflict of interests within families, both between people of different gender and different age.

The attempt at resolving the dilemma, which the discourse appears to recognise, that is, that of the criticism of social workers for being both insufficiently vigilant and/or overzealous, is achieved by suggesting a form of intervention which appears to be simultaneously supportive of both children and parents. However this is mythical in three important respects. In the first place, the interests of the children and the parents may not coincide. Second, there may well be conflicting interests, because of power differentials, between parents. Third, the notion of the family in play in the discourse appears to be that of the nuclear family with two parents. It should be remembered that many of subjects/objects of social-work intervention are single-parent families.

Recommendations

The Committee of Inquiry makes a number of recommendations and the more important ones are briefly summarised later. The discourse of the Report in this section can again be seen to be attempting to resolve the dilemma considered above by asserting the equal importance of both children and their 'parents'. This is illustrated by considering the recommendations in relation to both children and parents.

Children

Perhaps the most widely quoted recommendation in relation to children is

> There is a danger that in looking to the welfare of children believed to be victims of sexual abuse the children themselves may be overlooked. The child is a person and not an object of concern.
>
> (p. 245)

The way the Report seeks to realise the ambition to treat the child as a person and not an 'object of concern' is to explain to children what is going on, and to offer explanations as to why they are being removed from home. They should also be given a clear idea of what is going to happen to them, and promises should not be made to a child which cannot be kept (p. 245).

Professionals are also urged to listen to children and to take seriously what they say. Also the views and wishes of the child, particularly as to what is going to happen to them, should be taken into consideration, and they should be placed before any court dealing with the case. The Committee does not suggest, however, that 'these wishes should predominate' (p. 245).

The Report suggests that children should not be repeatedly medically examined purely for the purposes of evidence, and their consent should be obtained for such examinations and for photography. Neither should the child be subjected to repeated interviews of a 'probing' nor 'confrontational' type, and consent should be obtained before the recording of interviews on video. Furthermore, medical examination should take place in a 'suitable and sensitive environment' by 'suitably trained staff' (see pp. 245–6).

Parents

The Committee of Inquiry recommend that parents of children who may have been sexually abused be accorded the same courtesy as the family of any other referred child, that is, they should be kept fully informed and be consulted, if appropriate, at all stages of an investigation. Parents are 'entitled to know what is going on' (p. 246). All decisions should be confirmed in writing by the Social Services Department, in order that they may, if they wish, take legal advice about any particular decision. Parents should be advised of their right to appeal and complain, and they should be offered support by Social Services throughout the investigation. They should not be left 'isolated and bewildered at this difficult time' (p. 246).

Inter-agency cooperation

This is by far the largest section of this part of the Report. However, since this chapter will consider extracts from *Working Together – Under the 1989 Children Act – A guide to arrangements for inter-agency co-operation for the protection of children from abuse* (Department of Health 1991), which has become the official discourse in relation to inter-agency cooperation, it is appropriate to focus simply on the first recommendation of the Report. The first recommendation is of major significance because while it insists that no single agency has 'pre-eminent responsibility' for the assessment of child abuse and child sexual abuse, nevertheless the statutory duty of Social Service Departments must be recognised. This is crucial since it must remain the case that for all the envisaged and very important inter-agency cooperation, the recommendation nevertheless does not envisage a change in the basis of statutory duty, and it is precisely this duty which centralises social workers in the problem of child abuse.

The importance of this lies in the fact that whatever criticisms may legitimately be made of the Cleveland Social Services Department in terms of the management of the cases in question, it is nevertheless clear that they acted in pursuance of their statutory duties. Nowhere in the Report, or in any other quarter, has it been suggested that they acted illegally; insensitively at times, perhaps, but nevertheless within a legal framework of statutory duty. The Place of Safety order was the then-existing emergency provision for the protection of children from abuse. It was not the prime responsibility of the Social Services Department to secure convictions, but to protect the child.

The removal of a child from home is a trauma for the child and also for any non-abusing parent or caretaker in the household, that is, overwhelmingly mothers. The abuser or alleged abuser in such a situation may remain in the comfort of his own home. Therefore, it is now common to attempt to remove where possible the alleged abuser and not the child. The social-work policy is then to attempt to support the 'non-abusing family network'.

As is illustrated earlier, there is discretion available in terms of the way in which a statutory duty is pursued; however, the statutory duty remains. It should also be borne in mind that in Cleveland there was an unprecedented number of children diagnosed as victims of sexual abuse over, in the main, a 2-month period. This could easily stretch the coping capacities of the most sensitive of Social Service Departments.

It could be asked, therefore, whether even a policy such as that outlined earlier would survive such a crisis. There are serious resource questions involved in attempting to keep over 150 children at home when they have been diagnosed as victims of sexual abuse, and the Social Services Department, their preferred policy notwithstanding, may have been forced to managerially resort to Place of Safety orders in order to fulfil their statutory duty.

Perhaps we should also consider what might have been said in a subsequent public inquiry had Cleveland attempted to keep the children at home only for them to be diagnosed as suffering further abuse as a result of that, despite the best efforts of their social workers to support the 'non-abusing family network' and to remove the abuser from the child's home.

The discretion involved in such cases, therefore, takes place within specific statutory parameters is underpinned by the discursive and ideological roots of these parameters. Essentially it is a choice between, on the one hand, familialism (even if in some cases of a modified form, e.g. it may involve the recognition of the changing family household form, or it may recognise that a part of a 'family', i.e. an abusing member of the household, or extended family household network, is a danger to a child) and, on the other hand, a specific statutory intervention to protect and remove the child.

The difficulty that Social Service Departments and their staff face, or certainly faced, under the law as it existed at the time is to anticipate in advance what is the right emphasis between the above two parameters – that is, preventing the removal of the child, and statutory intervention to remove the child – before knowing what will be the final outcome.

For there to be a Public Inquiry there has to be an outcome which is unintended, protested or otherwise regarded as wrong by a sufficient number of people, and which is drawn to the attention of the Secretary of State. In other words it is often only via the hindsight of an undesirable final outcome that agencies and their staff find themselves under critical scrutiny. Where there is discretion between two parameters that are necessarily at times in tension and even in direct conflict, there has to be a judgement, and this is a judgement not about proof beyond all reasonable doubt, but a judgement concerning the balance of probabilities. There will therefore be times periodically and inevitably when a social worker and her/his agency gets it wrong, and this is not surprising, even if it is often tragic. The discourse contained within the report attempts to resolve this dilemma by asserting the importance of the rights of both children and parents, and by suggesting a form of intervention, which promotes a form of familialism. This version of familialism, further developed in the 1989 Children Act, glides over the difficulties and contradictions involved in that concept.

It therefore remains necessary to consider the changes brought about by the 1989 Children Act, and the White Paper upon which the Act is based, which is entitled *The Law on Child Care and Family Services*. The White Paper itself arose from a report on children in care by a House of Commons Select Committee which reported in July 1985. The Government responded by setting up a working party, which published a consultative document in September 1985 which was entitled *Review of Child Care Law*.

Ungendered subjects in the discourse of familialism

It is of significance that when the White Paper informs a reader of the objectives of the proposed changes in the law, parents and children appear as ungendered subjects:

> In bringing forward these proposals for change the intention has been to achieve greater clarity to help parents and children who may be affected by the law... The other prime objective has been to seek improvements in the law so as to offer a fairer deal to both children and parents.
>
> (p. 1)

This is important because it is overwhelmingly if not exclusively the case that the children who were the subjects of recent public inquiries, and who were subject to physical abuse, sexual abuse, and murder, were girls and the perpetrators men. As David (1991) points out:

> In the inquiries, however, what was the key issue was not the intergenerational gender relationship but the inter-generational relationship per se, with mothers receiving as much critical attention as the perpetrators of the abuse.
>
> (p. 113)

The reason for this non-recognition of gendered subjects lies in the strong familialism which is clear and explicit in the White Paper. This becomes particularly clear when the principles of the proposed Act are outlined. It is worth quoting from the first three:

a.   the prime responsibility for the upbringing of children rests with parents. The State should be ready to help parents to discharge that responsibility especially where doing so lessens the risk of family breakdown;

b.   services to families in need of help should be arranged in a voluntary partnership with the parents ... ;

c.   the transfer to the local authority of parents' legal powers and responsibilities for caring for a child should only be done by a full court hearing following due legal process.

There are a number of points which should be noticed here. There is the explicitly stated intention to locate the upbringing of children with 'parents'. However, this is not couched in terms of a right; rather it is posed as a question of responsibility. Perhaps where there is a right the question of intervening into, or even removing, that right is more complex than intervening where a 'parent' is seen as not fulfilling a responsibility. Also if one has a right to parent a child at home then one might have a right to call upon the State for help in upholding that right. However, if one has a responsibility to care for the child then to call upon State assistance necessarily involves one in the admission of at best difficulty in, and at worst failure in fulfilling that responsibility; and this is despite the protestation of the discourse to the contrary (see later), since the feelings of those who are subject to and subjects of the discourse will not change simply on account of the stated intentions of the discourse.

The White Paper announces the intention to create a 'better balance' between the State and individual parents. The reader is informed that the Review of Child Care Law listed 'three themes on which more emphasis is placed nowadays' (p. 3). These three themes can be summarised as: involving children and parents in decisions about services provided for them; recognising that parents are often the true contestants of court proceedings affecting their child; and that there needs to be a 'clearer acknowledgement' that in care proceedings the aim is to 'get the right result for the child', and that the procedures and representation should 'be better directed to this end' (p. 3).

This is immediately followed by the recommendation that the Place of Safety order lasting for 28 days 'no longer seems appropriate'. The 1989

Children Act substitutes for this an Emergency Protection order which lasts for only 8 days with a provision for one 7-day extension. The order can be applied for by anyone, to a court or to a magistrate. A court must be satisfied that the child will suffer 'significant harm' if it is not removed to accommodation provided by the applicant, or if the child does not remain where it is, for example, if the child is in hospital (see section 44 (1) (a), Children Act 1989), or that an investigation of a risk of significant harm is being frustrated by an unreasonable refusal of access (see section 44 (1) (a), Children Act 1989). This order can be challenged 72 hours after it is made, by anyone with parental responsibility or anyone with whom the child was living when the order was made.

The endeavour to maintain separate interests for the child

The White Paper explicitly contests the view expressed by 'some respondents to the Review of Child Care Law' that the proposals would 'shift the balance too far towards the interest of the parents and away from the interests of the child' (p. 2). The White Paper insists that

> That belief is misplaced. A number of changes proposed in the law would provide greater protection than at present for the child. These include the power to take action to prevent future harm to the child, and a 'best interests of the child' test in deciding whether to return a child home who is subject to a care order.
>
> (p. 3)

The White Paper also indicates that there are strong arguments in favour of a family court. However, the Paper itself concentrates on proposals which seek 'to improve the effectiveness of magistrates' courts' procedures in the kinds of cases at issue' (p. 3). In fact the 1989 Children Act did introduce a number of new courts. They are Youth Court which replaces the Juvenile Court, which deals exclusively with criminal matters and which now extends to young people up to the age of 17 years, and a Family Proceedings Court in which serves magistrates from a specially trained panel.

Services to families with children

Chapter 2 of the White Paper is entitled 'Services to Families with Children'. In this chapter it is proposed that local authorities be given a 'broad umbrella power' to provide services to children and families which 'promote the upbringing and care of children' and prevent 'family breakdown' (p. 4). This power is to be utilised to provide services to children and parents both at home and, if necessary, in residential accommodation. Financial assistance is something, however, that the local authority is empowered to provide only in 'exceptional circumstances' (p. 5). This provision illustrates the way in which the particular form of familialism in the Act is of an authoritarian nature. The government insist that 'families' offer the best environment in which to bring up children, and parents have a responsibility to look after them – services will be provided for those in need – however, only in exceptional circumstances will financial assistance be provided. Hence the government expect 'families' to care for children, and they will provide 'services', for example a social worker, but little or no money. Nevertheless if parents fail in this responsibility the State will intervene. For instance, the White Paper also envisages that the duty 'under current legislation' to receive children into their care in 'specified circumstances' will remain, but

> Such a service should, in appropriate circumstances, be seen as a positive response to the needs of families and not as a mark of failure either on the part of the family or of the professionals and others working to support them. An essential characteristic of this service should be its voluntary character, that is it should be based on continuing parental agreement and operate as far as possible on a basis of partnership and co-operation between the local authority and parents.
>
> (p. 5)

In order to underline this change of emphasis the document proposes that local authorities should no longer be 'under an obligation' to diminish the need to receive children into their care on a voluntary basis. This, the White Paper suggests, underlines the positive aspects involved in the idea of promoting the upbringing of children by families. However, the same paragraph states that the duty to diminish the need to receive children into their care, where necessary, on a compulsory basis via a court order should remain (p. 5).

The document also calls for the abolition of the then existing provision whereby parents wishing to remove a child from voluntary care must give 28 days' notice. If the authority cannot agree with the request, because they feel that the child will suffer harm as a result, then they must resort to an Emergency Protection order. Neither will the local authority have resort to a 'parental rights resolution'; it may, however, 'reserve the right to withdraw their services to child and family; similarly the parent can withhold or withdraw the child' (p. 6). A local authority could also apply for a Care Order under the grounds proposed by the White Paper, and which appear in the Act, which are specified in section 31 of the Act, and are that a child up to its seventeenth birthday, or sixteenth if married, is suffering or is likely to suffer 'significant harm' attributable to the care given, or likely to be given to the child, and in addition not being what it would be reasonable to expect a parent to give her or him, or the child is beyond parental control. The court must also be satisfied that making such an order is better than making no order at all.

All of the above is related to the provision of support and services at a general level to families. This section of the White Paper translates in the Children Act 1989 into the following general duty which is specified in section 17 of the Act:

> L.A. has a general duty to safeguard and promote welfare of children 'in need' and, so far as is consistent with that duty, to promote their upbringing by the families by providing a range and level of services appropriate to their needs.
>
> (Smith 1991: 8)

A child is said to be 'in need' if

> She/he is unlikely to achieve or maintain, or have the opportunity to so do, a reasonable standard of health or development without provision of services by an L.A.; or health and development likely to be significantly impaired, or further impaired, without such services; or is disabled.
>
> (Smith 1991: 8)

To all of this should be added the duty to reduce the need for care proceedings which is specified in Schedule 2, paragraph 7 of the Act. The local authority (LA) must take reasonable steps to reduce Care/criminal/family proceedings leading to Care. It must also avoid the need for Secure Accommodation, and encourage children not to commit crime. In addition the provision under Schedule 2, paragraph 4 of the Act is that the 'L.A. shall take all reasonable steps through the provision of Family Support services to prevent children within their area suffering ill treatment or neglect' (Smith 1991: 10).

Familialism and the dilemmas for social workers

The White Paper and the Act place emphasis on a positive notion of family support; there is now a specific duty to promote the upbringing of children in 'families', that is, by people with 'parental responsibility'. Parenting is couched in terms of a responsibility and not a right. Nevertheless the duty of an LA is to work in partnership with parents. In other words, they must always work where possible and where appropriate with parental agreement etc. This is certainly a stronger emphasis than that existing in earlier legislation. There is also a duty to prevent 'significant harm, neglect', etc., and to diminish the need for compulsory care proceedings.

The public enquiry that has been considered earlier in relation to the events in Cleveland was a situation in which the duties to prevent, protect, rehabilitate, etc. were in clear conflict. Is there reason to believe that the Act, containing as it does a stronger duty to 'keep families together' and to provide non-compulsory services to children 'in need', and yet which does not diminish in any way the duty to instigate investigation and proceedings where there exists concern that a child may come to significant harm, will simplify matters? On the contrary, there will remain periodically, episodically but inevitably, the crucial times where the line between prevention, protection or rehabilitation will remain so fine that it may only be fully visible with hindsight. This will become yet clearer when the discourse of the White Paper in relation to children at risk is considered.

Children at risk – a more active duty

Chapter 4 of the White Paper is entitled 'Protection of Children at Risk'. The second paragraph indicates that there has been 'particular public concern derived from some recent tragic cases of child abuse' (p. 11). The White Paper points to the Jasmine Beckford case and the subsequent Panel of Inquiry Report, 'A Child in Trust'. It suggests that the Government has taken this and other reports 'into consideration in assessing whether this aspect of the law can be improved' (p. 11).

Immediately following that paragraph a reader is informed that it is proposed to instigate a 'more active investigative duty' than that which exists under the then current legislation. Hence, the LA is now under a stronger obligation to investigate. It is very difficult to overcome the dilemma outlined earlier. The situation now obtaining is in essence that there is a stronger inducement to face in two conflicting directions, that is a stronger duty to keep families together and a stronger inducement to investigate situations in which they could or should be separated. This is easy to say and difficult to do. There will be times when social workers will be actively promoting togetherness when perhaps they should be actively investigating separation, as in the Maria Colwell case and other subsequent cases like it, for example, Jasmine Beckford; or, alternatively, they will be actively investigating separation when perhaps they should be actively promoting togetherness, as was alleged in some at least of the Cleveland cases and subsequent cases like them. Social workers could not be blamed for thinking that they were in a 'no win' situation in relation to work with children and families.

Inter-agency cooperation – a solution to the dilemma?

In the Cleveland inquiry, much was made of the lack of inter-agency cooperation even though, as is outlined earlier, communication between particular agencies broke down because of fundamental differences of attitude and belief reinforced by, in the case of the police and the Social Services Department, differential requirements of proof. A further question to be considered therefore is whether the issue of inter-agency cooperation can in some way ameliorate the problem. The White Paper outlines the proposals on this issue as follows:

> The Jasmine Beckford Report declared that there were powerful reasons why the duty on local authorities or health authorities to co-operate...should in the context of child abuse be made more specific, to include the duty to assist by advice and the supply of information so as to help in the management of such cases.
>
> (p. 11)

The White Paper argues that such a statutory duty would promote inter-disciplinary work both in the investigative stages and in terms of follow-up action. It tells a reader that the Government 'accepts this view' (p. 11). The White Paper's proposal on inter-agency cooperation translates into section 27 of the Act which indicates that 'there is a mutual obligation on Authorities to assist one another unless there is conflict with their own statutory duties' (Smith 1991: 8).

Working together

It is surely worth posing the question as to the extent to which such a provision may have helped matters in Cleveland. It is the case, as is indicated earlier, that the LA social service departments are, in fact, further centralised in the issue of child abuse. Only they (and the NSPCC) can bring care proceedings; they have a more active investigative duty, and also a duty which is at best in tension with, and at worst conflicting with, that of promoting the upbringing of children with 'families'. This is a very different duty than that of the police whose primary duty is to detect crime and secure a conviction. Where there are both differential attitudes to a problem, and differential duties in relation to a problem, then inevitably there will be at least tension and perhaps, in times of perceived crisis, open conflict. This is at least a part of the explanation for the events in Cleveland. However, the above tensions are apparently not noticed by the authors and bearers of the discourses within British childcare legislation. It is as if all would be well if only the differing agencies had the will and capacity to 'work together'.

It remains therefore to consider some extracts from the document *Working Together – A guide to arrangements for inter-agency cooperation for the protection of children from abuse* (Department of Health 1991). The document was produced by the Home Office, the Department of Health, the Department of Education and Science and the Welsh Office.

The centrepiece of inter-agency cooperation was envisaged as the area child-protection committee, and the document states that 'There needs to be a joint forum for developing, monitoring and reviewing child protection policies. This forum is the Area Child Protection Committee (ACPC)' (p. 5).

A reader is also informed that ACPC members are accountable to the agencies that they represent (membership being drawn from all agencies with an involvement in child protection), and the agencies are 'jointly responsible' for ACPC actions. Furthermore, 'the individual agencies should endorse the policies, procedures and actions of ACPC' (p. 5).

It should be recalled that in Cleveland there was in existence such a committee. However, it seems that the total circumstances obtaining at the time of the crisis produced a situation where relations between two agencies broke down to the point of each one going its own way. Such a crisis is an exceptional circumstance, as are all child-abuse cases which ultimately become the subject of public inquiry. Perhaps it is true that improved inter-agency cooperation, joint work and joint training will help in routine cases, or even more complex cases, but the issues involved in the relatively few, though important cases, in which there are tragic results can always 'break the back' of such arrangements. This is particularly important when there are differing roles, functions and statutory duties, and when one agency has both the 'lead role' *and* functions and statutory obligations which themselves may be in tension or even conflict.

Part 4 of the document specifies the role of agencies involved in child protection. Since the role of the LA Social Service Department has been outlined already in the present chapter it is appropriate to focus briefly on the role of the police. Significantly the document recognises that

> Police involvement in cases of child abuse stems from their primary responsibilities to protect the community and to bring offenders to justice. In the spirit of *Working Together* the police focus will be to determine whether an offence has been committed, to identify the person or persons responsible and to secure the best possible evidence in order that appropriate consideration can be given to whether criminal proceedings should be instituted.
>
> (p. 16)

The document also recognises the tension that exists between the differing statutory duties of both the police and the Social Services Department. The document continues:

> Difficulties will be encountered in joint inter-agency investigations but these can be minimised by the selection of specialist staff who undergo appropriate inter-agency training…. It is important that those engaged in child abuse investigation and their supervisors fully understand the responsibilities of both agencies, the powers available to them and the different standards of proof that exist in relation to criminal and civil proceedings. This will assist to remove some of the tension that can otherwise exist.
>
> (p. 17)

The document does not claim that the tension which 'can otherwise exist' will be eliminated, merely that the proposal will assist in removing some of it. The question thus remains of how much of the tension will be removed by this recommendation and, crucially, in what circumstances might such tension resurface? Perhaps in a situation like Cleveland where doctors act in good faith and make a diagnosis of sexual abuse, which the police believe will not secure a conviction, but the Social Services nevertheless, in pursuance of their statutory duty and having a lesser burden of proof, that is, the evidential requirement of a civil court, feel obliged to act. It will also be true that under the Act they will be under a stronger obligation to do so.

On the other hand, a potential situation could be envisaged whereby all the agencies on the ACPC agreed that there was insufficient proof of abuse, on either criminal or civil grounds, yet there was still concern, but the parent or parents would not agree to the child's being 'looked after' on a voluntary basis by the local authority. In this situation, the Social Services in the 'lead role' would be attempting to promote the upbringing of the child or children by the 'family' while attempting to carefully monitor the situation. Other agencies that had experienced inter-agency training could be involved and information could be shared, but none of this entails that mistakes, deception, misconception and miscommunication could not sometimes occur, and it may well do so with tragic consequences.

Joint training and the inadequacy of instrumental reason

The document under consideration devotes a section (Part 7) to the question of joint training. In the introduction to that section the document specifies what it envisages as some of the content of that joint training and it adopts an extremely instrumental tone – skills and knowledge are key requirements. This is because

> Effective child protection depends not only on reliable and accepted systems of co-operation, but also on the skills, knowledge and judgement of all staff working with children in relation to child protection matters. It is important therefore that people in direct contact with children receive training to raise their awareness of the predisposing factors, signs and symptoms and local procedures relating to all child abuse matters.
>
> (p. 53)

There is, unfortunately, an immediate and significant problem with this. It concerns quite simply the question of the *existence* of skills and knowledge in the areas in which the document assumes it. The question has to be posed as to where this knowledge, upon which to base a skilled intervention, exists. For such knowledge one would turn to academic texts and research on the subject. Unfortunately, however important this may be, it is nevertheless not made easy by the fact that there is little or no consensus in the literature as to even the definition of abuse, the extent of abuse or the typology of abusers. There is also the question as to the importance of the various ways of conceptualising the problem – historically, socially and politically, etc. – and all in the context of the time available to agencies, and to social-work training courses, etc., to impart such skills and knowledge.

The discourse under consideration glides over all of this and reassures a reader that the kind of catastrophes to which the discourse is in part a response can be resolved, or greatly minimised, by interagency cooperation and joint training. However, the centrality of the social worker, together with the unacknowledged problem of the statutory duties that they are obliged to carry out, which often may be in tension or outright conflict, and which are even more strongly re-emphasised in the 1989 Children Act, remain as a discursively constructed tightrope which, periodically, episodically and inevitably, social workers will be unable to walk.

The documents which have been the focus of this chapter promote, as has been argued and illustrated earlier, a particular form of familialism. The issue of gender oppression within families appears not to be recognised. The 'family' is stripped of all gender; 'parents' are referred to, but rarely are mothers or fathers; children are referred to, but rarely little boys or little girls. These genderless 'parents' have an obligation to bring up genderless children, and services in the form of social workers and other welfare professionals will be provided, but only in exceptional circumstances will these involve money. Social Service Departments are placed under both an obligation to work in partnership with 'parents' but are also under a stronger duty to investigate them if they believe that their children are at risk of 'significant harm'.

The documents are strongly managerial, technical and instrumental in their approach. Ultimately it is a combination of inter-agency cooperation and knowledge and skill which is mobilised. In this sense the 1989 Children Act represents more of the same. The various documents that have been considered in this chapter have placed their faith in various knowledges and practices. What is lacking is any recognition of the limits of such knowledges and practices. The remainder of the book will illustrate ways in which social workers, as they currently exist, are themselves, in significant part, a creation of the discourses and ideologies which will be considered in the remaining chapters. Hence each chapter will argue that they have been centralised within successive legislation and faced with a task which is at best very hard to fulfil, and at worst impossible without the use of hindsight. The State itself, together with the many academic texts considered in this book, has consistently failed to recognise the fact that a central problem is the massive difficulty of the task itself. The remainder of the book illustrates that the Children Act 1989 is no exception. In fact by further centralising Social Service Departments into the 'lead role' and imposing a stronger duty to investigate, together with a duty to work in partnership with parents, it represents an amplification of the dilemma which concerns this book. The following chapters therefore consider the historical emergence of these discourses and ideologies before returning to the question of how all of this impacts upon contemporary social-work practice.

Chapter 5

A stitch in time

The men from the ministry

This chapter considers some of the discourses and ideologies contributing to two Acts of Parliament. They are the Children and Young Persons Act 1933 (HMSO 1933), and the Children Act 1948. In pursuit of this the chapter considers the work of the Children's Branch of the Home Office in the 1920s and 1930s and the emergence in those official circles of a discourse of prevention. Hence the chapter attempts via the scrutiny of the Home Office Reports on the Work of the Children's Branch of 1923, 1925, 1939 and also the Report of the Departmental Committee on Sexual Offences Against Children and Young Persons 1925, and the 1927 Departmental Committee on the Treatment of Young Offenders, to uncover the emergence of this discourse. It then briefly considers the Curtis Committee of 1945–6, both the final Report and the interim Report, which calls for training in childcare and suggests its form, content and duration. The chapter argues that all of this provides a better appreciation of the post-war period in terms of the development of professional state social work in Britain, and the construction of subsequent childcare legislation, than that which is on offer in the various social-work texts cited in the chapter.

SOCIAL-WORK TEXTS AND THE 1933 ACT

It is important to consider social-work texts which, in so far as they focus upon the 1933 Act at all, do so briefly but all nevertheless seem to take the view of the 'standard' social history on the subject, which appears to suggest that the Act is transitional between rescue/rehabilitation and prevention/treatment. Hence it is of importance that this period be carefully considered.

There are a number of problems with this sort of analysis. Foremost among them is that, in ignoring the period between the passing of the 1908 Children Act and the period up to the 1927 Department Committee on the Treatment of Young Offenders, one can be left imagining that a significant shift had taken place, or was at that time taking place, and rather a mysterious one at that, since very little is on offer by way of explanation. It appears to be either the steady march of progress in the more 'standard' social-history version, or the generalised reactionary nature of the ruling class in the 'radical' versions. This is illustrated by comparing two recent social-work texts on the subject with the 'standard' social-history text, that is, Heywood (1978 – first edition 1953).

Two social-work texts which focus upon a history of child abuse or child welfare both present themselves as an analysis of the politics of child abuse and child welfare. Given that focus, a reader approaching these two texts might expect to find some in-depth analysis of the 1933 Act. Unfortunately that is not only not the case, but it is also true that these texts rely very heavily indeed on the 'standard' social history for the little that they do offer on the subject; for instance, Parton (1985) contents himself with quoting Heywood (1978)

> Although the emphasis on rehabilitation of the child is forward looking, the concept of care is still nineteenth century, based on removal from degrading environmental conditions of squalor and poverty, and provides substitute family for the home which has failed.
>
> (Heywood 1978: 130)

Heywood also suggests that

> The Act is memorable in setting a standard of welfare and rehabilitation for the delinquent and the neglected children and those in need of care which had never previously been approached. Ideas and philosophies which had required treatment of social failures and problems to be justified by hard work and stigma were now finally discarded and a constructive concept of social training in the best interests of the child took its place. The welfare of the child, and not the judgement of society was now paramount.
>
> (Heywood 1978: 130)

The fact that in the case of the 1933 Act Parton does not look beyond Heywood is further illustrated when Heywood suggests that 'the problem called not for caseworkers, but for policy of economic support for the family expressed in legislation' (Heywood 1978: 131), and apparently in turn Parton suggests that 'the alternative to the more authoritative rescue approach would have been the development of greater economic support for the family' (Parton 1985: 40).

Frost and Stein (1989), in one of the two paragraphs that they give to the 1933 Children and Young Persons Act, simply say that

> The main provisions of the 1933 Act were directed at the removal of the child albeit to 'reformed' or 'regulated' institutions or foster parents, and were justified by the new 'progressive' welfare ideology. It was therefore essentially a reactionary measure with no vision of prevention or indeed a return to a 'rehabilitated' family. It was an Act which gave expression to the ruling class forces of the day. In the face of massive unemployment, ill health and poor housing, child neglect was seen primarily as a product of 'bad families' from which children should be removed.
>
> (p. 32)

A greater depth than that offered by either of the two social-work texts encountered so far is required.

THE 1933 CHILDREN AND YOUNG PERSONS ACT

The 1933 Children and Young Persons Act was a consolidating Act. Its main focus was on 'infant life protection and juvenile delinquency'. It also contained a provision in relation to the control of young people: that is, as defined by the Act, people between the age of 14 and 17. The Act merged the Industrial Schools and the Reformatory Schools and gave them the title 'Approved Schools'. In a further linguistic transformation the words 'trial' and 'sentence' were eliminated from the proceedings of the juvenile courts. The Act also extended to 17 the age of young people coming before the juvenile courts and introduced the 'welfare principle' into the proceedings. Justices for the courts were to be selected for the court on the basis of their interest and experience.

The LA in the form of the Education Department was charged, by the Act, with the responsibility of providing information to the court about the young person before it, that is, family background, schooling, etc., and the LA was to have primary responsibility for bring children and young people before the court who were in need of 'care' and 'protection'. There was also provision for placing children and young people under supervision by a probation officer. These recommendations came from two main sources, and they were the 1925 Departmental Committee on Sexual Offences against Young People, and the 1927 Departmental Committee on the Treatment of Young Offenders. Both of these Committees appear to have been greatly influenced by the various reports of the Home Office Children's Branch which was founded in 1913 and which itself was formed as a result of a Committee of Inquiry set up to investigate the allegations of extreme cruelty, and a death, at the Akbar Nautical Training School in 1910.

The men from the ministry

Clarke (1985) offers a short and helpful history of the Children's Branch in this period, and he details some of the ways in which a centralising and professionalising strategy was adopted by the reformers at the head of the Children's Branch. He does not, however, consider very fully the impact that all of this had on the 1933 Act, nor does he illustrate in his own text that he is working extensively from the text of the reports of the Children's Branch of the Home Office in this period, since no direct quotations appear.

The function of the Children's Branch of the Home Office included the inspection of Reformatory and Industrial Schools. However, even a cursory glance illustrates that the brief was interpreted very proactively. Consider for instance this extract from the report of 1923 in which a reader is informed that 'opportunity has also been taken to include information on other matters which directly or indirectly concern young persons and which fall within the administration of the same Branch of the Home Office' (p. 4).

The authors of the report are adopting a proactive remit, and a reading of the various reports illustrates that they also have an agenda. It appears that the agenda is one of 'modernising', centralising, and standardising existing provision for the young offender. However it is also concerned with investigation and the generation of knowledge and resultant innovation, that is, the generation of new provision. Hence recommendations are made on a variety of issues. Ultimately what emerges is a discourse which looks towards training and treatment and away from punishment.

Causes of delinquency

The causes of delinquency in the eyes of the Children's Branch, in so far as they had a theory at all, appear to be lack of supervision and youthful high spirits combined with poverty. Consider for instance this extract from the same report of 1923 in which it is suggested that the

> Causes which lead to the commission of offences are no doubt as varied as the offences themselves, and it would be wrong to assume that boys and girls who appear in the Juvenile Courts come from criminal homes.... It is not found as a general rule that the homes from which these children come are hopelessly bad, and in a large number of cases the parents though very poor are decent and respectable members of the working-class. The same spirit of mischief and adventure is found in children of all classes of the community, but those from the poorer homes are in many instances not under adequate control or have not sufficient opportunities for giving proper expression to their energies. Poverty seems to be undoubtedly at the bottom of much of the delinquency among children.
>
> (pp. 4–5)

The report explicitly sets its face against heredity as being a main cause of delinquency, and the reason for this is clear and explicit: to do otherwise would, from the point of view of those who wish to offer training and treatment as opposed to punishment, produce too pessimistic a scenario. Hence the report insists that too much importance must not be attached to heredity as an excuse for wrongdoing. In the preface to a book recently issued the Dean of St Paul's wittily said, 'A good heredity will triumph over the most conscientious education.' Those who do not believe firmly in the converse proposition, that careful training can overcome even the serious handicap of a bad heredity, are not likely to be successful workers in the field of child welfare (p. 9).

Care, control and gender

The 1923 report makes a clear distinction between the problem of the youthful male offender and that of the youthful female offender. The report, in commenting upon the increase in juvenile crime during the period of the 1914–18 war rejects the theory that the problem is caused by the absence of fathers, at war, and therefore unavailable for the purposes of control and discipline, since the argument cannot be sustained statistically. The effect of the war was nevertheless given a causal role, but that causal role differs in relation to boys and girls. It is suggested that

> The nation was passing through a period of restlessness and excitement and the martial spirit of the boys was aroused. Many of the

legitimate outlets for unexpended energy were no longer available, because lads' clubs, boys' brigade, and boy scouts had lost their leaders ... the boys sought in vain for some means of satisfying their desire for excitement. Naturally a neglected baker's cart became a German convoy, the little gang a British patrol, and the loaves trophies of the raid. Much of the so-called crime was not in itself serious, but persistent mischief and misguided adventure are apt to have a demoralising influence. The younger girls were not so great a source of anxiety as the boys, *but for the older girls the conditions arising out of the War presented peculiar temptations owing to the lowering standards of morality, and too often it was found that the girls who came before the Juvenile Courts had dipped deeply and tragically into the* life *of the streets.*

(p. 10, my emphasis)

This view was to have further implications. The Report of the Departmental Committee on Sexual Offences Against Young Persons 1925 (HMSO 1925a) recommended that 'a parent or guardian shall have power under section 59 to charge a young person with being beyond control' (p. 74). This was an extension of the provision in the 1908 Act in that under that Act this power did not exist beyond the age of 14, and, though the provision applies to both boys and girls, nevertheless the reason for the recommendation is explicit concern about the control of the sexuality of adolescent girls. The section of the Report of the Departmental Committee on Sexual Offences against Young Persons in which this recommendation is made is headed 'Methods of Control (Adolescents)' and it states that 'We have evidence that many instances in which young persons between 14 and 16 have begun to lead an undisciplined life, and have defied every good influence brought to bear on them' (p. 73) and further suggests that

Witnesses of varied experience have brought to our notice that there is an increase in the number of young girls who are beyond control, and who are living in a manner likely to lead to their downfall, and they have urged that there should be power to deal with such cases under the Children Act by appropriate measures of protection. We have had instances reported to us in which girls have been misconducting themselves for over a year, staying out late at night and defying every measure taken to restrain them.

(p. 72)

The section points to a case 1894 in which a girl under 16 was found guilty of aiding and abetting and inciting a man to have 'unlawful carnal knowledge of her', but which was overturned on appeal since the Act under which she was tried did not intend that the girls for whose protection it was passed should be punishable under it for offences 'committed upon themselves'. The concern then was how to control the behaviour of adolescent girls, while being unable to use the charge of 'aiding and abetting', and also being unwilling to wait until the girl was charged with an offence in the juvenile court. It was for this reason that the 'beyond control' recommendation was made. Hence the Committee members

> Recommend that a parent or guardian shall have power under section 59 to charge a young person with being beyond control. We further recommend that machinery be devised for strengthening the Children Act to enable steps to be taken to protect young persons, boys and girls, who are out of hand, or who lack proper guardianship, by enabling them to be dealt with as beyond control.
>
> (p. 74)

Knowledge and power

The 1923 Report of the Children's Branch (HMSO 1923) is explicit concerning the need for knowledge of the child to be before the magistrates because

> It is generally recognised that to enable magistrates to arrive at a decision in any individual case... it is necessary for the magistrate to have full and complete information as to the child's record at school and as to the circumstances of his home.
>
> (p. 11)

The report goes on to suggest that a Probation Officer or School Attendance Officer should produce a full report while the child is on remand. Medical knowledge is also explicitly called for, and indeed it is suggested that the juvenile court should have at its disposal a doctor with 'experience of the mental as well as the physical qualities of children' (p. 12). In what is an interesting and important passage, developments in psychoanalysis are anticipated, since the report speculates that

> If it is true, as certain psychological writers have recently said, that the hypothesis of the unconscious motive is one of the greatest

discoveries of modern science, a great deal of light may eventually be thrown on the conditions which lead children to commit offences, and on the right methods of dealing with them. Even if the claims advanced by psychoanalysis...prove to be extravagant all who are responsible for the care of children must acknowledge renewed stimulus thereby given to the subject of child study which is likely to lead to more enlightened handling of young people by parents, teachers and others.

(p. 12)

Observation, assessment and expertise

The Report of the Departmental Committee on Young Offenders 1927 (HMSO 1927) develops the above and lays the ground for the foundation of what later became known as Observation and Assessment Centres. Under a section entitled 'Bail and Remand' the report suggests that 'in the more serious cases, however...some method has to be adopted for securing his reappearance or for the purposes of enquiry and observation' (p. 40).

However, when it comes to the elaboration of the above, it becomes clear that securing a reappearance is not the first and foremost item on the agenda since, after a brief resumé of the law on remand as it then stood, the Committee members indicate that they

> Have been much impressed by the views expressed to us as to the need of much greater facilities for the examination and assessment of young offenders. To the court is entrusted the very important function of deciding the right treatment to be applied to each particular case. Once the principle is admitted that the duty of the court is not so much to punish for the offence as to readjust the offender to the community, the need for accurate diagnosis of the circumstances and motives which influenced the offence becomes apparent.

(p. 43)

The remand in custody here is in the main for observation, assessment, enquiry, etc. The terminology is already medical, for example, 'examination', 'diagnosis', 'treatment', and it rapidly becomes clear that a medicalised space is being carved out, since the reader is immediately informed that

> More important still is the need for estimating the personal factors, including especially mental and physical health. There is always the

possibility of mental deficiency, the discovery of which would lead to special treatment.

(p. 43)

The report goes on to suggest that this examination and observation be available, where necessary, for all people under the age of 21 and that it should be available for the adult court as well as the juvenile court. This, it was thought, would be a great advantage since it would be possible to employ the same expert staff The Committee members add that the 'institutions should in our opinion be provided and maintained by the State and controlled by it' (p. 55).

If there is any residual doubt that the body and soul of the young delinquent is being passed to the control of the technical expert, this ought to be settled when the Committee finally suggests that 'matters of detail can best be settled by experts when Parliamentary sanction has been obtained for the scheme' (p. 45).

Linguistic transformation

The Committee also recommends a change of language in relation to the juvenile court. It suggests that 'the terms "conviction and sentence" should not be used in the juvenile court' (p. 122).

Such transformations may have a significance beyond even the authors' conscious intentions. However, it appears, in this particular case, that the authors are consciously mobilising such linguistic transformation. Their reasons for making this particular recommendation are outlined in a paragraph on page 32 of the report. The first reason given is that the Committee was 'constantly informed that young offenders suffer in after life as a result of a conviction by a court' (p. 32). The second reason is that the Committee sees 'no value in the use of the word "conviction" in juvenile courts and its disappearance would tend to mark the distinction between these courts and adult court' (p. 32).

There are a number of points which could be made in relation to this. In the first place it should be noticed that the words conviction and sentence, whatever other connotations they may have, also have a certain relational value, that is, they specify a particular relationship between participants in a process. The process is a judicial one in which evidence is presented, pleas are entered and guilt or innocence is recorded. The social gulf between the judge and the judged is massive and the power difference between the two is transparent.

The Committee members say themselves, and quite emphatically, that 'we are under no illusion that a change of name can be effectively used to conceal a fact' (p. 32), but nevertheless this does not prevent them from making the recommendation, and by causing the disappearance of these words they also cause the disappearance of their negative relational connotations. This then serves as an affirmation of the distinction between the juvenile and the adult court. If, as a result, employers are more willing to exploit the labour of the young people who become the objects of the interventions of the juvenile court, then that is all well and good, since all of this is part of the shift away from punishment. No doubt the Committee was genuine in its desire not to bar young offenders from careers for which they were 'eminently suited' since, in the case of the young male offender this was very often a branch of the armed services.

There is, however, a further reason for this particular transformation, which is not explicitly given in the text. It is the simple fact that a move away from punishment and towards treatment requires ultimately a large degree of discretion for the court in relation to the question of 'disposal'. The word 'sentence', coming as it does from the discourse of classical jurisprudence, implies proportional punishment. In other words a defendant is tried, found guilty and punished accordingly. The sentence has a fixed relationship to the crime. When it comes to treatment, however, this approach is insufficiently related to the particular individual before the court. Hence in the same paragraph in which the Committee gives its explicit reasons for the change of language, it reveals a less explicit but rather more important reason. The Committee suggests that 'when a child or young person is found to have committed an offence it should have power to make such orders as is suitable to the case, whether it be probation, guardianship, residential school or other treatment' (p. 32).

Sentenced to treatment

Under a section of the report headed 'Methods of Treatment' (p. 47), it becomes transparent that the report is creating a space for judicial discretion in the treatment of young offenders, since, before offering detailed recommendations, the Committee feels the need to 'make some general observations on this part of our inquiry'. They immediately suggest that

> At one time the attention of the courts was mainly confined to their primary duty of deciding whether the defendant committed the

offence alleged against him. The subsequent treatment of the offender received far less consideration. Indeed the choice of method was so restricted that little room was left for any exercise of discretion on the part of the judicial authority.

(p. 47)

What is taking place here is the prising open of a very particular kind of space. It is a space in judicial proceedings for medical knowledge. It is this kind of knowledge that the Committee is envisaging will be mobilised in advising the judiciary *how* to use the discretion that is being advocated. When this level of power is being sought, then the stakes are high, and when the stakes are high the potential return on them must be at least as high. In this particular case what is placed at stake is 'the whole question of crime'. This fact becomes clear when the Committee suggests that

> If there is any risk in making the assumption that most criminals begin their careers by committing minor offences, there is certainly evidence for the statement that a considerable number of them appear at an early age before the juvenile court. We may refer to the figures published in the Second Report of the Children's Branch, which show that of a thousand young men received into Borstal institutions no less than 551 committed their first offence before the age of 16, and many of them committed several offences before that age. *The juvenile court, therefore, by its wise treatment of the young people who appear before it must of necessity play an important part in relation to the whole question of crime.*

(p. 16, my emphasis)

What is implicitly offered here is the promise to significantly reduce all crime by the 'wise treatment' of juvenile crime. The words 'wise treatment' are loaded with a high degree of expressive value. Who would have any desire to treat young offenders unwisely? As is clear from the earlier, as the report unfolds, wise treatment becomes synonymous with what is essentially a version of medical treatment. Certainly the word treatment in the report takes on a relational connotation akin to that of doctor and patient. What is absent in the report is any fully fledged knowledge base to flesh out that relationship. The 'treatment' is essentially training, though the contribution of psychology and psychoanalysis is anticipated. Thus, treatment is presented as wisdom, as opposed to the unwisdom of punishment, which is its other.

This discourse is not passive, it is actively productive, nor is it tolerant of discourses which, as it were, stand in its way. The tone towards the discourse of punishment is ruthless indeed. Consider this:

> The acceptance of this principle may sometimes involve the substitution of a longer period of detention under skilled instruction for a short term of penal discipline. 'Five years in a reformatory for stealing two shillings' is the headline. The idea of the tariff for the offence or of making the punishment fit the crime dies hard; but it must be uprooted if reformation rather than punishment is to be – as it should be for young offenders – the guiding principle.
>
> (p. 48)

The metaphor mobilised is a harsh one, the discourse of punishment with its proportional tariff, etc., 'dies hard', that is, in this context insufficiently quickly, and therefore it must be 'uprooted'. If a tree is uprooted it surely dies and it does so quickly, furthermore after a while it rots and leaves no visible trace of itself. If, on the other hand, it is merely chopped down then, even if it dies, it will do so more slowly and its roots will remain for some time. Furthermore, what is in this context worse, it may grow new shoots and that would never do, since there is a new plant growing in its place which is to be the 'guiding principle', that is, the discourse of reformation/training/treatment.

This chapter began with quotes suggesting either that the 1933 Children Act could be seen as transitional between, on the one hand, a 'forward looking' concept of 'rehabilitation' and a nineteenth-century concept of care based on the simple removal of children from 'conditions of squalor and poverty' (Heywood 1978) or, on the other hand, which simply dismiss the 1933 Act as 'a reactionary measure' giving expression to the 'ruling class forces of the day' (Frost and Stein 1989). These conceptions of the matter do not offer sufficient depth. A closer examination of the various texts cited thus far in the chapter appears to show that a very specific 'discursive struggle' is taking place. It is essentially the struggle of the discourse of treatment against that of punishment; the former has to be 'uprooted' if the latter is to take its place.

Poverty is acknowledged, given the period it could hardly not be, but the discourse nevertheless, for all that, in no way recognises that a response to this problem can be any part of a solution to juvenile crime. On the contrary, it calls instead for greater supervision and greater training. It must of necessity significantly discount heredity since not to do so would risk leaving the field open to the biologist, and not to the trainer or the educator. It is the subjectivity of the young offender which has to be penetrated and influenced. The raw material is, in the main, young people from homes whose parents are very poor but nevertheless 'decent and respectable members of the working class'.

The men from the ministry, in the form of the Children's Branch of the Home Office, had, by the time of the 1933 Children and Young Persons Act, carved out the social space within which the technical 'expert' would begin to operate, and within which s/he would ultimately flourish, if never finally actually triumph over the competition from the legal expert.

This has implications for the analysis offered by the social-work texts cited and criticised earlier, and especially so when it comes to considering their view of subsequent Acts, and perhaps particularly the 1948 Act. The problem is that the 'technical expert' had been at work for far longer than these texts appear to recognise. The texts in question therefore place too much store (or blame) upon the Labour Government of 1945 for the creation of the 1948 Act. This can be illustrated by taking the clearest case first, which is undoubtedly that of Frost and Stein (1989). We are told, for instance, in relation to the 1948 Children Act that

> The experience of mass unemployment of the 1930s and the means testing of poor relief meant that the labour movement was determined to bring about forms of welfare that did not stigmatise, divide and humiliate.
>
> (p. 33)

They immediately continue by suggesting that

> The spirit of 1945 and Labour's social democratic politics provided the ideological climate for the acceptance of welfare policies which reflected a more liberal and humane approach, *a significant break with policies, practices and theories that had gone before*.
>
> (p. 33, my emphasis)

Hence in the space of less than two pages we have moved from the 1933 Act as a 'reactionary measure...which gave expression to the ruling class forces of the day' (p. 32), to the 1948 Act as reflecting 'a more liberal and humane approach' and constituting a 'significant break' (p. 34).

This account gives too much agency in the process to the Labour Government. It appears to suggest that the 'significant break' is essentially the result of this Labour Government. It is almost as if the Labour Government and the expert arrived together, or even that the Labour Government ushered in the expert. However, when it is realised that the expert had already been in place for over 20 years, working in the Home Office Children's Branch, constructing what perhaps to him (or her) was a more humane discourse, and a more scientific discourse, that is, that of treatment as opposed to punishment, then this notion of a significant break dissolves, and with it dissolves the idea of a Labour Government in 1945 entering government, in this context, as a new broom sweeping all before it.

The process was infinitely more complex. Who recruited whom? Did the Labour Government recruit the experts? Or, did the experts recruit the Labour Government? More the latter than the former perhaps, but equally, no doubt, since the Labour Government was committed to reform, it gave the experts their head. On the other hand it is not clear that these experts would not have had their head if another government had been in power.

It is helpful at this stage therefore to take as a starting point the continuing discourse of the Home Office Children's Branch, in order to fill in some of the space between the 1933 and 1948 Act.

Report of the Children's Branch 1938

There are three important points which a consideration of this report (HMSO 1938) illustrates. In order of appearance in the report they are: (1) the fact that in relation to the 'care and control' provisions of the 1933 Act it has already become the case that older girls are more numerous than older boys in relation to being subject to this provision; (2) a theory of delinquency and deprivation located within the concept of the 'broken home' appears; and (3) the discourse, while still being the medical discourse of treatment, moves into the modality of prevention. They can now be considered in their order of appearance.

Care and control

In chapter 8 of the report, which is entitled 'In Need of Protection, or Beyond Parental Control' the care and control provision is introduced by suggesting that

There have been cases before the courts in which it has been represented by an anxious mother that her daughter of 16 was beyond her control and in which it has been found by the court that the mother was attempting to enforce a degree of control over her daughter which was quite unreasonable. The not unnatural disinclination of a daughter to submit to what she regards as excessive parental domination is sometimes hotly and bitterly resented by the mother as unnatural filial disobedience. A case occurred, for example, in which a girl of nearly 17 working as a shop assistant was only allowed to retain a minute fraction of her wages, was expected to economise on lunch if she took a bus to work and was never allowed to go to the cinema except when she was chaperoned.

(p. 38)

This is the pattern of the examples throughout the report: that is, although the provisions apply to both boys and girls, all the examples provided concern older girls. When it comes also to the gender and age distribution of the young people against whom this provision was used, the gendered nature at the upper-age range is very clear indeed. The report informs a reader that

There follows therefore the interesting conclusion that about 330 boys and 400 girls over 14 have been dealt with under the new Act with whom it would not have been possible to deal with under the previous Act. It also appears (as was to be expected) that the number of older girls is larger than the number of older boys, the reason being that amongst the older girls there are to be found a greater number in a state of emotional adolescent instability, than among the older boys.

(pp. 39–40)

There are a number of important things to notice in the aforementioned. First among them is the fact that within the discourse of treatment there is now in place a notion of 'emotional adolescent instability'. It can be criticised in and of itself, but it is also important to consider its specific mobilisation in this particular discourse. Readers of this report might find themselves wondering, apart from what a state of 'emotional adolescent instability' actually is, why older girls are apparently more prone to fall victim to it than older boys. Taking the latter question first, the answer becomes clear less than one page later when a reader is informed that

Included amongst the girls who come within the innocent description of being 'in need of care and protection' are some of the most difficult cases with which the juvenile courts and the approved schools have to deal, girls who are in a state of emotional, adolescent disturbance, impatient of control and used to a large measure of liberty and licence.

(p. 41)

It is interesting that the provisions themselves are described as innocent. The concept of innocence here is used to contrast with a (female sexual) other of innocence which is meshed within the provisions for the 'most difficult cases'.

There is more to be said about this; indeed it could be the basis of an entirely separate book, but it appears in this chapter because the texts that are considered within it do not appear to notice this unfolding either and it is clearly important. It is important also to notice, as it were, where it starts. As well as illustrating the gendered nature of these provisions it also illustrates that a medical/psychological concept of adolescence was by now being produced and mobilised. Girls are more likely than boys to suffer from 'emotional instability' as a result of it, which manifests itself in the girls' being in 'moral danger'.

The earlier is also important because it serves to further illustrate that the experts and the medical/psychological discourse which they produced did not have the good grace to wait for a Labour victory before taking the stage. This point becomes much clearer and is best developed when it comes to further considering the 1938 Report of the Home Office Children's Branch, and hence this chapter now moves to another section of that report.

Broken homes

In chapter 9 of the report, entitled 'The Approved Schools', in the space of five pages there is concentrated a theory of delinquency, and an argument for its prevention. It should be considered in some detail. The chapter opens with the claim that the record of the Approved Schools had been one of 'steady and substantial progress'. The close cooperation and collaboration existing between the juvenile courts, the Home Office and the managers of the schools is declared to be important in

straightening out the lives of many thousands of young people whose *early environment has encouraged*, if it has not actually caused, the commission of offences against the law, or *whose neglect has been such as to make an early lapse probable, if not inevitable.*

(p. 42, my emphasis)

This small paragraph is very concentrated indeed. There are several important things to notice in this passage. Resisting the temptation to comment on the very instrumental metaphor of 'straightening out', the use of the term 'early environment', which is given a strong determining role in delinquency, can be highlighted instead. Delinquency is also explicitly linked with neglect. Neglect is a specific case of an early environment. As becomes clear as the discourse unfolds, the distinction being made in this paragraph is essentially the distinction between being *deprived* in early environment and having a *depraved* early environment. However, both are seen as having the same consequences. Those consequences are that while a depraved early environment encourages, if it does not cause, delinquency. On the other hand, a deprived background makes delinquency probable, if not inevitable. In other words, both a *depraved* early environment and a *deprived* early environment lead to delinquency. Either by encouraging it, or causing it, they make it probable or inevitable. It is important to remember this because it illustrates that the foundations of much later reforms were being laid here, and laid much earlier than is often recognised.

For instance Frost and Stein (1989), writing about the much later Ingleby Committee and the Children and Young Persons Act of 1963, suggest that

> First, the Report made the link between delinquency and family neglect. The disturbed family came to be seen as the key to both deprivation and depravation. The conflation of these two concepts is the key to understanding the eventual passage of the Children and Young Persons Act 1969.
>
> (p. 36)

While Pitts (1988), discussing the 1965 White Paper entitled *The Child, the Family and the Young Offender*, suggests that conventional criminology complained that the proposals it contained

> involved an unjustifiable lumping together of the deprived with the depraved, which would stigmatise and corrupt the poor but virtuous by thrusting them into close association with the feckless and the delinquent.
>
> (p. 13)

Prevention

The truth of the proposition that this period, that is, the mid-1960s, represented the high-water mark of the discourse of treatment, or that this conflation of the deprived with depraved did not take place at the time that the authors quoted earlier suggest is not in question here. Nevertheless, it is important to notice that the discourse can be found virtually fully formed, nearly 30 years earlier. This makes the 'triumph' of the discourse a slower, more incremental process, than is implicitly implied in the texts quoted earlier.

This is illustrated further by considering the next few passages in the 1938 Home Office Report. Under the heading 'The Problem' a reader is given a pen picture of

> The young hooligan seeking adventure, the lad who has perhaps been unemployed for months and drifted into a dishonest life, the adolescent girl, restless, seeking escape from a humdrum life or uncongenial employment and finding it through immoral conduct, and the boy with a real or imaginary grievance against the community – these form the problems which the schools have to face.
>
> (p. 42)

The temptation to be resisted here is to dwell upon the seemingly ever present double standard in which female misconduct is always apparently sexual, and sexual conduct from a boy is never a matter worthy of mention. Not because this is not important, it is, but the passage immediately following this pen picture puts it into a context – a very clear causal context, and this is very important in analysing the discourse. A reader is informed that these boys and girls have often been

> described as the failures of our educational system, but it would be more correct to attribute their downfall to the unsatisfactory social conditions which unfortunately still exist in London and in our great industrial areas, for it is from these that the children of the approved school are mainly gathered.
>
> (p. 43)

However, the focus immediately shifts from unsatisfactory social conditions back to the education system, or more concretely, to illiteracy through truancy. The Report suggests that some of this illiteracy is a result of

> A limited brain power, but in too many instances, it has been their cleverness, if not their intelligence, which has enabled them, no doubt with the connivance of their parents, to evade the activities of the school attendance officer.
>
> (p. 43)

But nevertheless the numbers of these young people in relation to the general school population are declared to be negligible, and hence it becomes possible to characterise them as 'misfits', since

> The success of these young people in avoiding attendance at school in these days when the attractiveness of elementary school education has diminished truancy to an almost negligible quantity is only an indication of the failure of our social system to pick up these misfits and find a remedy at an early age before their character and conduct have become problems for the juvenile court.
>
> (p. 43)

There is a characteristic slide taking place here. It is the slide from, on the one hand, social conditions as in an important sense causal, that is, an analysis which would lead to an interrogation of the social system with a view to changing it, to, on the other hand, a social system which is failing a few 'misfits'. It is allegedly doing so by failing to identify these 'misfits' at an early age, before they have become 'misfits' – thus recognising the alleged fact that, at a later age, they will become misfits – and doing something, we know not what, about it, before it is too late. This leaves the social system, that is, the social whole, the totality, unexamined; hence, any causal role that it may have goes unrecognised – acknowledged yes, recognised no.

All of this produces the shift to the individual subjectivities of working-class youth – boys and girls differentially, that must surely by now be clear – but to the subjectivities of the poor, working-class young, nevertheless. Not just to some of them, but potentially to all of them, since the discourse is now essentially about prevention and therefore necessarily prediction, and however flawed an enterprise and tall an order this may be, it must involve some level of potential surveillance and therefore intrusion into all of the subjectivities of working-class youth.

The Report having made its plea for prevention is then driven by its own logic to the question of prediction, or in its own language, 'predisposing causes'. Hence a reader learns that

> Writers on the problem of juvenile delinquency have called attention to the effect of 'broken home' – one of unhappy parental relationships, illegitimacy, and similar conditions as pre-disposing causes, particularly in the case of girls.
>
> (p. 43)

It is interesting to note that the discourse here does not dwell on the particular claimed cause. Admittedly it gives it a great deal of space and it does not question it, and there are questions that could be, and no doubt ought to be posed, for example, is correlation the same thing as cause? But the discourse is impatient to move on; the problem is not so much that these young people had to suffer for several years their bad early environment – their 'broken home', etc. – which troubles the Home Office. It is rather that this early environment causes later delinquency, and if it is (probably) necessary to change this environment then it must be done sooner and not later. Again we have prevention – prevention via prediction – because, if intervention into 'broken homes' is called for prior to the committal of an offence, in order to prevent one, then this intervention is necessarily an intervention into all 'broken homes' since quite clearly there is no way of knowing in advance which 'broken homes' out of all of them will produce the delinquency, unless of course they all do.

What appears to be taking place is that there is a move within the discourse of treatment from cure to prevention, that is, from the removal and rehabilitation of children in the 1920s, which was the view which held sway when the 1933 Act was introduced, to early identification of predisposition, that is, prediction and prevention by 1938, a view which was a decade later to inform the 1948 Act.

An examination of the 1938 Report of the Children's Branch of the Home Office suggests that the emergence of the discourse which was to inform the 1948 Act was a smoother, more gradual, more incremental, and altogether more evolutionary affair than seems to be suggested by the short accounts in the texts that are criticised earlier. The discourse simply does not contain the twists, turns or even 'U' turns that would be necessary to grant one permission to see the 1933 Act as in some important way reflecting the 'reactionary' wishes of the 'ruling class' and the 1948 Act as reflecting the 'liberal, humane' aspirations of the working class as represented by a Labour government. The British State is in itself more continuous than is suggested by this. The men from the ministry have their own strategy and momentum which can, and in this particular case did, survive relatively unscathed, despite changes of government.

When it is realised, for instance, that a Mr A. H. Norris, a former medical inspector with the Children's Branch, was at the head of the Children's Branch from 1917 up to and including 1938 and was therefore (of course) the 'obedient servant' of a number of Home Secretaries, inclusive of those of a Conservative government, a Labour government, a National government and of another Conservative government again, the importance of his particular discourse becomes clear. Furthermore, an examination of his discourse through this 21-year period gives no indication that he, and therefore it, took any great account of these varying 'masters', to whom he remained, always and ever, of course, the 'obedient servant'.

THE 1948 CHILDREN ACT

It is appropriate in the light of the above to move to outline and analyse the discourse of the Curtis Committee which was very instrumental in the production of the 1948 HMSO Children Act. This is important because, apart from anything else, it is the production of the 1948 Children Act which, according to at least two authorities, establishes a fully fledged 'modern' system of individualised social service. Consider for instance Leeding, who suggests that

> In general terms child care may be defined as a blend of legislation and practice which inspires the social care of children and young people under the age of 18. It has a long history, but the modern concept developed after the Second World War when the Curtis Committee report was followed by the Children Act of 1948, which for the first time established a social service specifically for children who for various reasons were unable to live with their parents under normal home conditions. This service led inevitably but gradually to a concern for the families of such children.
>
> (Leeding 1976: 1)

The matter is put even more clearly by Bolger *et al.* (1981: 86) when they say that 'the 1948 Children Act differentiates itself from ... nineteenth-century social policy by looking at the individualised needs of each child and by constructing a specialised and individualised serviced based on these needs'.

The Curtis Committee and the 1948 Act

The Curtis Committee was appointed in March 1945. Its terms of reference were

> To enquire into existing methods of providing for children who from loss of parents or from any cause whatever are deprived of

a normal home life with their own parents or relatives; and to consider that further measures should be taken to ensure that these children are brought up under conditions best calculated to compensate them for the lack of parental care.

(Curtis Committee: A3)

It is important to notice that these terms of reference do not concern children living at home, in however miserable conditions. The Committee considered the care of children who for 'any cause whatever' were already removed from a 'normal home life'. There is a clear reason for this. The Curtis Committee was called into being as a result of the death of a 7-year-old boy named Dennis O'Neill, who was 'boarded out' to the care of foster parents. There was an inquiry into the specific circumstances of the tragedy but the government had, in addition, ordered that the general situation be considered and this resulted in the setting up of, in the case of England and Wales, the Curtis Committee.

There is a paradox involved in all of this. Dennis O'Neill died as a result of ill-treatment by his foster father. It was nevertheless the Committee's strongly expressed view that where a child could not be maintained at home then, where possible, such a child should be fostered. This paradox was perhaps an important moment in the ultimate residualisation of residential childcare.

Children's homes and familialism

A very strong concept of familialism is present in both the interim report and the report itself, expressed through the strong and no doubt accurate criticisms that the Committee members had of the institutional provision that they found upon their many visits to nurseries, children's homes and workhouses. There are two responses to finding unsatisfactory conditions prevailing within children's homes, etc. One is to conclude that they should only ever be used as a last resort, and the other is to say that they could and should be made much better. After all, the Committee was called into being as a result of the death by mistreatment of a child in *foster care*, not the death of a child in nursery care, a children's home or even a workhouse. The report essentially constructs the hierarchy of natural family, substitute family, children's home, etc. The report suggests that, where possible, children's homes should be smaller. There should be small 'family group homes', in which there should be trained 'housemothers' and 'housefathers'.

Familialism and maternal deprivation

In reading the Curtis Report it seems that one is reading a discourse *within* a discourse. Consider, for instance, the following passage which suggests that 'the dangers of institutional life for children, even where the institution is well-managed, arise out of a tendency to a lack of interest in the child as an individual and to remote and impersonal relations' (p. 160).

The same paragraph suggests that in physical terms – food, clothing, accommodation, etc. – children in 'Homes' are better cared for. However all of this serves to contrast with what is lacking on the 'human emotional side'. The Committee members have become convinced by what they tell a reader that they have seen themselves about such children, that is, that

> They continually feel the lack of affection and personal interest. The longing for caresses from strangers, so common among little children in Homes, is in striking and painful contrast to the behaviour of a normal child at the same age in his parents' home. The lack of a mother's fondling cannot be entirely made good, but something must be provided which gives the child the feeling that there is a secure and affectionate personal relation in his life.
>
> (p. 160)

The discourse within a discourse is that of maternal deprivation within the discourse of treatment. It is perhaps significant that the Committee not only came to the conclusions that it did come to via what its members saw, but also via what they heard from their witnesses. One of the witnesses was Lt Col John Bowlby, MD, RAMC, and another was Dr D. W. Winnicott, MRCS, MRCP, and yet another was Dr A. H. Norris, CBE, MC, MRCS, LRCP, DPH, formerly Chief Inspector, Children's Branch, Home Office. Of course there were many other witnesses, but these three are clearly quite a powerful and significant trio. This chapter has already considered the importance of the discourse of Mr Norris, and while limitation of time and space precludes a full examination of either Bowlby or Winnicott, it is important to at least offer sight of it, if only to indicate its 'fit' into the recommendations of the Curtis Committee. It has an obvious utility in the context of the discourse of treatment and of its material deployment in the legislation under consideration, and this is what is meant by the suggestion that reading the Curtis Committee report is like reading a discourse within a discourse.

It is as if, in a sense, the discourse of maternal deprivation rides 'piggy back' on the discourse of treatment.

It is necessary at this point to sound a word of caution. It is often asserted that versions of psychoanalysis with a strong focus on early mother and child interaction led very directly to, and always and every-where served as, a discourse/ideology through which the removal of large numbers of women from the workforce was legitimated in the immediate post-war period. However, as Riley (1983) suggests,

> certainly the general spirit of Bowlbyism in Britain in the mid1950s would have made the question of the provision of child care for working mothers almost unaskable – but this is quite a different proposition from putting the events of 1945 down to psychology and psychoanalysis.

(p. 116)

She continues in her chapter to trace a story of inter-departmental rivalry in the government and also the very important role of regional difference within the immediately post-war economy, all of which led to differing and uneven outcomes on this issue. Her work is valuable because it illustrates that too much store can be set by ideology or discourse or other subjective phenomena in assigning to it too great a determining role.

For instance, Mitchell (1975: 228) is quoted in Frost and Stein (1989: 35), whom they suggest captures this change of role in her passage when she informs her readers that

> Instead of national workers they were to be private wives... in the effort to rebuild the family the equation went: delinquent = latch key kid = having been abandoned by its mother in infancy to crèche or evacuation. From now onwards appeals to maternal guilt vied with the political exploitation of the economic situation to keep women at home... we learned that a person sucked his emotional stability literally with his mother's milk.

The analysis on offer here assumes too much of a seamless glide facilitated by a discourse/ideology. It appears to give it too great and too complete a determining role. This is not the same thing as saying that it had no determining role, or that it was not powerful. Indeed its power can be illustrated by considering even briefly the discourse of both John Bowlby and David Winnicott.

In now therefore turning briefly to Bowlby and then equally briefly to Winnicott, the concern is not with the truth claims of their particular discourse or even with interrogating its construction. The project is more simple and more mundane. It is simply to give an indicator of its power and of its strength in the immediate post-war context. This is important because, perhaps, the strength and power of this discourse in its context gives the clue as to why there was such a full-blooded lurch into familialism. After all, as is indicated earlier, Dennis O'Neill did not die in an institution, he died at the hands of foster parents, but so strong is the discourse that the paradox is not recognised – it is apparently not even worthy of comment, yet it is surely a paradox.

Writing in the preface of a later work and *recollecting the times in question*, John Bowlby, who served as an Army psychiatrist and who later, from 1946 to 1969, was the Director of the Department of Children and Parents at the Tavistock Institute for Human Relations, acknowledges a debt to a colleague, James Robertson. Robertson had joined Bowlby in 1948 and had brought with him accounts and files of children suffering from 'maternal deprivation'. Bowlby had already been 'struck' by the wide measure of agreement in 'regard to both the principles underlying the mental health of children and the practices by which it may be safeguarded' (Bowlby 1978: 12). Hence in his report for the World Health Organisation in 1950 he proposed that 'what is believed to be essential for mental health is that the infant and young child should experience a warm, intimate and continuous relationship with his mother (or permanent mother substitute) in which both find satisfaction and enjoyment' (p. 12).

Just in case a mother reading the book was still thinking of dropping Johnny to the nursery, she ought perhaps to bear in mind that 'the young child's hunger for his mother's love and presence is as great as his hunger for food . . . absence inevitably generates a powerful sense of loss and anger' (p. 13). Should she persist it may be that the following few, well-chosen words from Dr Winnicott (who, while he was writing in 1971, nevertheless, in his preface, informs a reader that his book is a development of a paper he gave in 1951) may be of assistance, since

> There is no possibility whatever for an infant to proceed from the pleasure principle to the reality principle or towards and beyond primary identification (see Freud 1923) unless there is a good-enough mother (not necessarily the infant's own mother). The good-enough 'mother' is one who makes active adoption to the

infant's needs... success in infant care depends on the fact of *devotion*, not on cleverness or intellectual enlightenment.

(p. 11, my emphasis)

This devotion cannot go on forever. Children have to grow up; they cannot go on forever omnipotently imagining that their mothers are 100 per cent devoted to them. A child should not forever have the illusion that

> Its mother's breast is part of the infant... under the baby's magical control.... The mother's eventual task is to gradually disillusion the infant, *but she has no hope of success unless at first she has been able to give sufficient opportunity for illusion.*
>
> (p. 13, my emphasis)

The earlier powerful extracts are offered because they illustrate that the discourse in question is powerful. The trio of Bowlby, Winnicott and Norris was very powerful, and all of them gave evidence to the Curbs Committee.

There were powerful social and economic circumstances in evidence. The end of the war, the experience of evacuation, separations of adult women and men from their loved ones, the separation of children from parents and, no doubt, the climate created by a collective commitment to social justice that the Labour victory represented, helped this discourse within a discourse – that is, the discourse of maternal deprivation within the discourse of treatment – to hold sway in the way it did. It appeared, on the face of it, not to be repressive and it was constructed as a service. Nevertheless, for all that, it is by attention to the discourse itself, which was already in an important sense lying in wait for these circumstances – that is, in the sense that in its essentials it had already been constructed – that a fuller picture emerges. In the light of this picture the essential recommendations of the Curtis Report come as no great surprise. However, to outline them will further demonstrate the hold of the discourses under consideration.

Training in child care

The Committee produced the Interim Report (1946a) because 'at an early stage' in its investigation it became apparent that 'a large section of the staff caring for such children were without any special training for the task, and this circumstance was in part responsible for unsatisfactory standards where these existed' (Curtis Committee: A2).

The report is very brief. It contains only 9 pages and an appendix of a further 8 pages. The Committee's first recommendation is that a Central Council for Training in Child Care should be established, the functions of which would be to 'administer a scheme of training as prescribed in this report and such other schemes as may be added later' (p. A3). The training course proposed displayed a massive commitment to familialism. This is particularly clear when the duties of the trained childcare workers are outlined. For instance it is suggested that

> the House Mother or Assistant Matron should be a woman suitable to take charge of a 'family' group of up to 12 children from (say) 2 years of age to 14 or 15. She must play the part of a mother to the children and be able to create for them the atmosphere of affection and security necessary to their happiness.
>
> (p. 4)

It is a very tall order for a woman to play the part of a mother for up to a dozen children to whom she is in no way related, but this is nevertheless considered to be her task.

On the other hand the corresponding male worker

> must play the father's part. His duties call for an equal understanding of and interest in children but his domestic work will lie on the side of out-of-door and recreational activities rather than the physical care of the child.
>
> (p. 4)

The central theme of familialism, with a rigidly defined gendered role for men and women, is clear from the aforementioned. It is important to note the 'fit' here with discourses/theories/ideologies that assert the central importance of motherhood, and early experience in the family, in the context of a scientific commitment to treatment/prevention: that is, a discourse which essentially claims to be able to prevent delinquency via early individual intervention into the subjectivities of young working-class people. That psychoanalytically oriented theories of casework could come to occupy a position as the knowledge base of the social-work profession throughout the 1950s, 1960s and even much later is not surprising given this 'fit', and the social and economic circumstances in which these discourses/theories/ideologies first became articulated with each other.

When it comes to the recommendations in relation to the local authority the essential rationale is to end potential administrative confusion. The Committee points out that

> the local authority for one purpose, e.g. child life protection, may be different from the local authority for another purpose, e.g. public assistance. ... [and] this may lead to a position in which no one feels actively and personally responsible for the welfare of the individual child.... We consider that all the children without a normal home life coming within the central department's sphere in a particular area should be under the care of the county or county borough council, and under one committee of the council.
>
> (p. 144)

The Committee even points out that it has evidence of a large measure of agreement with this proposal, and also evidence that many local authorities are already 'moving in that direction' (see p. 144). They also point out that many of their witnesses made representations urging that the committee of the local authority carrying these responsibilities should not be the Public Assistance Committee, and here the question of stigma is raised. Hence the Committee ultimately favours an *ad hoc* committee drawn from members of the various other committees which at that time had various responsibilities for deprived children. The committee was, hardly surprisingly, to be called the *Children's Committee*. The setting up of a new committee with centralised responsibility gives additional strength to the recommendation that a Children's Officer of similar status to a Medical Officer of Health or Chief Education Officer be appointed to each Children's Committee or, where there would be an insufficient workload, jointly to a number of committees. She would (the Committee members 'use the feminine pronoun not with any aim of excluding men from these posts but because we think it may be found that the majority of persons suitable for the work are women'), be 'a specialist in child care' (p. 46), 'highly qualified academically, if possible a graduate who has also a social science diploma and should have experience of work with children' (p. 148).

While it is certainly true that the Curtis Committee was responsible for the extension of the scope of public care of children, and for the disengagement of that extended public care from the Poor Law through its recommendation for a centralisation of its functions at both a national and at a local level, under a Children's Officer, nevertheless there are important ways in which all of this was an extension of what was already taking place, or had already taken place. At the discursive level the die was cast in its essentials in 1938, and at the administrative level the break with the Poor Law was less of a break and more of a 'tidying up' than is appreciated by the social-work texts that have been considered in this chapter.

Chapter 6

The 1960s and the short-lived 'triumph' of treatment

The purpose of this chapter is to consider the legislation of this later period against the analysis outlined in Chapter 5. It does so by, throughout the chapter, critically considering the position that Bolger *et al.* (1981), Parton (1985), Frost and Stein (1989) and Pitts (1988) take in relation to the Ingleby Report, the Children and Young Persons Act of 1963 and the White Papers *The Child, the Family and the Young Offender* of 1965 (HMSO 1965) and *Children in Trouble* of 1968 (HMSO 1968). The chapter then analyses the discourse in all of these documents and considers it in relation to the view that this period represented the triumph of the discourse of treatment over that of punishment.

The chapter argues that, notwithstanding the fact that the 1960s represented the high-water mark of the discourse under consideration, it is nevertheless true that the texts which are considered set too much store by changes ushered in by reforming Labour governments.

It is also argued that the consequence of overstating the extent of the triumph of the discourse of treatment over that of punishment is that it overlooks the extent to which the former is firmly underpinned by the latter, while it remains nevertheless true that, in particular periods, one end of the dichotomy may appear in sharper relief than the other. The chapter is particularly critical of Parton (1985) for going so far as to suggest that in the 1960s 'it is almost as if it was assumed that a conflict of interests between child, parents and the state had disappeared and the nineteenth-century problems of cruelty and neglect had been virtually abolished' (Parton 1985: 45).

The chapter argues that this position cannot be maintained. Its essential fault line is that it overlooks the continuity of the discourse of both punishment and treatment, and its attendant discourses, in relation to childcare legislation in Britain. It also overlooks the continuity of the British state as a source and bearer for such discourses and it therefore falls prey to placing too great an emphasis on sudden breaks with past law, policy and practice. These breaks then only become explicable in relation to factors in operation at the given time, for example a reforming Labour government (Pitts 1988 on the 1969 Children and Young Persons Act), a radicalised working class (Frost and Stein 1989 on the 1948 Act) or, in a slightly later period, moral panic (Parton 1985 on the 1975 Children Act). Hence, the chapter offers a more detailed account of the period under consideration than that which is offered by the texts cited earlier.

THE INGLEBY REPORT AND THE CHILDREN AND YOUNG PERSONS ACT 1963

Bolger *et al.* (1981) suggest that

> The 1963 Children and Young Persons Act was very ambitious in its aims. The policy makers hoped to get children's departments to combat juvenile delinquency and promote the welfare of children by helping the family as a whole to function 'properly'.... The necessity of *preventive* work with families, was beginning to gain some credence.
>
> (p. 87, my emphasis)

It should be remembered in relation to the above that the question of prevention was an important issue in the Report of the Children's Branch as early as 1938, as quotes from that document in Chapter 5 illustrate, and to suggest that in 1963 the notion was only beginning to gain some credence, it seems to me, is to understate the matter, since it is clear that this notion already had credence within the British state.

It is also clear that, by 1954, social work is considered, at least by Clare Winnicott, as a highly skilled and professional activity requiring particular kinds of knowledge, since she suggests that

> Our professional relationship is in itself the basic technique, the one by means of which we relate ourselves to the individual and to the problem. But what of the professional self that relates? If we look at it objectively we find it is the most highly organised and integrated part of ourselves. It is the best of ourselves, and includes all our positive and constructive impulses and all our capacity for personal relationships and experiences organised together for a purpose – the

professional function which we have chosen. In other words, it is a function of the super ego, with which the ego has easily identified because it has evolved from loving identification with early parental figures.

(Winnicott 1984 [writing in 1954]: 11)

Clearly, social work had by this time, at least internally and in some quarters, a strong professional identity, notwithstanding the fact that the requirements of a 'professional' self seem exacting to say the least, especially given the rudimentary training and even more rudimentary pay that was envisaged by the Curtis Committee's interim report, *Training in Child Care*.

In relation to this issue, Frost and Stein (1989) seem, on this occasion, to be more accurate, recognising, for instance, that by the early 1950s, 'caseworkers were appointed to work with families in what became known as preventive work' (p. 36). They recognise also that by the mid-1950s 'this was an increasingly important area of the department's work' (p. 36). However, there was at that time no recognition of that fact in law. It was the Report of the Committee on Children and Young Persons (the Ingleby Report), which made the prevention of reception into care a statutory obligation. These authors say of the Ingleby Report (Ingleby Committee 1960) that in retrospect it was 'a watershed in terms of the State's legitimation of welfare ideology. Throughout the decade that followed the welfare model was to gain increasing influence and recognition within the central and local State' (p. 36).

Prevention/treatment and the 'white heat of technological revolution'

Pitts (1988), in relation to the Ingleby Report, suggests that

The issue of social class is always bubbling just beneath the surface of any serious discussion of juvenile crime. The Ingleby Committee... established in 1956 rediscovered this class connection.... Their report argued that delinquency might be an indicator of social deprivation and that this deprivation might be prevented by the infusion of welfare resources into neighbourhoods which produced high juvenile crime rates.

(p. 1)

He also points out that the report

> alerted us to another problem; an over emphasis on the social
> compensation of deprived offenders delivered, via the justice sys-
> tem, through the medium of welfare or treatment, might shade into
> a denial of the legal rights of the young offender. This important
> consideration was largely ignored in the subsequent debate within
> the Labour Party about the role and function of the juvenile court.
>
> (p. 2)

The point that Pitts is making here is that the 1965 White Paper, *The
Child, the Family and the Young Offender*, advocates the 'decriminalisation' of juvenile crime, and attempts therefore to dispense with any form
of trial, except where there was a dispute as to the facts of the case, in
other words where there is a 'not-guilty' plea. Witnesses appearing
before the Ingleby Committee had advocated such a system, and the
Ingleby Committee had found against it, presenting as its reason for so
doing the issue of a young person's right to judicial procedure.

In fact Pitts' central argument, in relation to the distinction between
the Ingleby Report of 1960 and the later *The Child, the Family and the
Young Offender*, turns on this question of decriminalisation which finds
expression in the latter report. This is of course understandable, because
if court proceedings can be dispensed with altogether – though in fact
this was not envisaged in cases where there was a dispute – then treatment will have finally and fully triumphed over punishment.

However, it appears that again there may be at work here a tendency
to overstate the change that was produced by a Labour government.
There are times when Pitts appears to be mesmerised by the rhetoric of
Harold Wilson who, in his speeches of the time, spoke of the 'white heat
of the technological revolution'. Perhaps Pitts overlooks the extent to
which this was a device to make the Labour Party appear 'modern' after
13 years of opposition. It was suggested in Chapter 5, for instance, that
the discourse of treatment versus punishment was far more developed
within the Home Office Children's Branch than some authors appear to
recognise, and this has led them seemingly consistently to grant too
great a degree of causality to the reforming enthusiasm of successive
Labour governments.

It seems reasonable to expect that if Pitts is correct in suggesting that
in 1964 Harold Wilson ushered in the 'eggheads' as 'righters of social
wrongs', and it was this that was the driving force for the alleged triumph of treatment, then there should be, 'Butskellism' notwithstanding,

a difference of significance between the Ingleby Report and *The Child, the Family and the Young Offender*, since they were produced by a Conservative government and a Labour government, respectively.

In the event the proposals in *The Child, the Family and the Young Offender* were withdrawn, and the Home Office Childcare Inspectorate, in the personage of Joan Cooper and Derek Morel, drew up instead the White Paper entitled *Children in Trouble* which was the compromise that formed the basis of the never fully implemented 1969 Children and Young Persons Act. Be that as it may, it remains fair to Pitts to compare Ingleby with *The Child, the Family and the Young Offender*, since it is the latter that represented what Labour wished to do, and hence that report is considered immediately below.

The Ingleby Report

The Ingleby Committee was appointed in 1956 with the following terms of reference:

> to inquire into and make recommendations on:
>
> (a)   the working of the law in England and Wales, relating to:
>
>> i) proceedings and the powers of the courts, in respect of juveniles brought before the courts as delinquent or as being in need of care and protection or beyond control;
>>
>> ii) the constitution, jurisdiction and procedure of juvenile courts;
>>
>> iii) the remand home, approved and approved probation home systems;
>>
>> iv) the prevention of cruelty to, and exposure to moral and physical danger of juveniles;
>
> and
>
> (b)   whether local authorities responsible for child care under the Children Act, 1948 in England and Wales should, taking into account action by voluntary organisations and the responsibilities of existing statutory services, be given new powers and duties to prevent and forestall the suffering of children through neglect in their own homes.
>
> (p. ii)

Chapter 1 of the report, entitled 'General Approach', confronts what it sees as the puzzle of juvenile delinquency. While the position in relation to the general problem of children in trouble, including those in need of care or protection and those suffering through neglect, is thought to be 'not altogether discouraging', there is nevertheless a problem in relation to the increased level of juvenile delinquency. What is thought to be not discouraging is that the stability of the family, 'badly shaken by the disruptions of war, and of the post-war period seemed to be improving' (p. 3). The indicator advanced to illustrate family stability is a decline in the number of maintenance and affiliation orders in 1956 as compared with 1947. The Report also sees cause for optimism in the fact that after the war 'the education and welfare services had been greatly expanded and were still developing' (p. 3).

Prevention/treatment and the post-war rise in juvenile delinquency

However, as regards delinquency, the Report concludes that while

> The sudden steep rise in the official figures in the mid thirties was thought to have been due largely to a greater willingness on the part of all concerned to prosecute under the Children and Young Persons Act of 1933, and not necessarily to indicate a real rise in juvenile crime. The further big rise in the figures during and since the war is more alarming, particularly as, in spite of fluctuations, they have remained well above the 1939 figures.
>
> (p. 3)

The Report continues its analysis of the figures, and it appears that the figures for 1958 dispense with any commitment to the theory that the disruption of the war and the resulting instability of the family and the absent father was the problem. This is because

> Fifteen years after the end of the war far from improving, the situation is more serious than it has ever been. In view of this it is not possible any longer to feel sure that in spite of the temporary setback of the war years our methods of dealing with children in trouble (whether actually delinquent or not) are generally sound and efficient and necessarily developing along the right lines. We have therefore felt it necessary to reconsider our approach to the whole question.
>
> (p. 4)

This reconsideration of the whole question turns in the discourse on the question of cure versus prevention. The Report quotes from the

Report of the Committee on the Treatment of Young Offenders (HMSO 1927) which, while focused on methods of cure rather than prevention, nevertheless had no doubt of the wisdom of the old proverb 'Prevention is better than cure'. This further illustrates the sense in which the discourse of treatment and prevention versus punishment unfolded in a more incremental way than is often recognised.

The Committee's terms of reference included the issue of the working of the law in England and Wales relating to 'the prevention of cruelty to, and exposure to moral and physical danger of juveniles' and of whether local authorities should be 'given new powers to prevent and forestall the suffering of children through neglect in their own home' (p. 1). The Committee therefore reports that the extract of its terms of reference above had inevitably led it to consider the 'efficacy of the existing preventive influence' (p. 5). However, the committee is determined to be positive and productive. For instance they indicate that they

> Have found it impossible to consider the question of prevention from a purely negative point of view. It is not enough to protect children from neglect even if the term neglect be held to include their exposure to any physical, mental or moral danger or deprivation...something positive is required. Everything within reason must be done to ensure not only that children are not neglected but that they get the best upbringing possible.
>
> (p. 5)

Familialism is, as one might expect, central to the idea of 'the best upbringing possible'. The Report immediately continues to speak of the duties of parents and the duty of the community. The duty of parents is to

> Help their children to become effective and law abiding citizens by example and training and by providing a stable and secure family background in which they can develop satisfactorily. Anything which falls short of this can be said to constitute neglect in the widest sense, though obviously the degree of such neglect which can justify interference by a court must be more rigidly defined.
>
> (pp. 5–6)

It is the fact that parents are said to vary in their capacities to perform these duties, and the fact that children vary in the extent to which they present problems to their parents, which calls forth the 'duty of the community' (by which they mean the State) which is

> To provide through its social and welfare services the advice which such parents and children need; to build up their capacity for responsibility, and to enable them to fulfil their proper role. In considering the second part of our terms of reference (namely whether local authorities responsible for child care should be given new powers and duties to prevent children suffering from neglect in their own homes), we have had this positive aspect of the problem constantly in mind.
>
> (p. 6)

What the discourse is beginning to put in place here is selectivity, the 'community' (the State) has a 'duty' to provide services for the minority of parents and children who are, for one reason or another, unable to conform to 'recognised standards of behaviour' (p. 6).

The puzzle of delinquency and neglect and its causes remains the subject material of chapter 1 of the Report. The committee settles for the 'reasonable possibility' that such delinquency and neglect is a result of 'a lack of a satisfactory family life' (p. 7). This is because the experience gained by 'all those working' in the newly expanded welfare services, such as

> social workers, psychologists, psychiatrists and others is invaluable, and has materially effected the outlook on the question of how to bring up children.... It is the situation and the relationships within the family which seem to be responsible for many children being in trouble, whether the trouble is called delinquency or anything else.
>
> (p. 7)

The report points out that only 2 per cent of those 'children at risk' have to be dealt with by the court as offenders in 1 year. It then suggests that no

> complete explanation can be given why this two percent get into trouble while the remaining ninety-eight percent do not, but it seems a reasonable possibility that one of the factors leading to the failure of this two per cent has been the lack of a satisfactory family life.
>
> (p. 7)

Clearly there is a large degree of circularity taking place here; correlation is not the same thing as cause. It was already the dominant 'knowledge' base of the profession that the family was in one way or another central, and the very legislation which gave the various workers in the field the power to intervene was influenced by the same familialism. It is as if, in a closed circuit, the discourse provides the evidence for the discourse. To a significant extent the bearers (and developers and originators) of the discourse in the field, inform the bearers (and developers and originators) on the Committee of Inquiry. The discourse appears to feed upon itself.

A 'material, moral and social revolution' and the construction of the problem family

The Report also considers what it calls 'wider influences', by which it means influences beyond the family. It appears compelled to do this because the steepest reported rise in juvenile delinquency is in the older age groups, that is, 14–16-year-olds and 17–21-year-olds, and it can be argued that young people, as they grow older, become progressively less influenced by the family, but more influenced by 'other environmental and cultural influences' (p. 7). The report continues by suggesting that

> While life has in many ways become easier and more secure the whole future of mankind may seem frighteningly uncertain. Everyday life may be less of a struggle...but the fundamental insecurity remains with little the individual can do about it. The material revolution is plain to see. At one and the same time it has provided more desirable objects, greater opportunities for acquiring them illegally, and considerable chances of immunity from the undesirable consequences of so doing. It is not always so clearly recognised what a complete change there has been in social and personal relationships (between classes, between the sexes and between individuals) and also in the basic assumptions which regulate behaviour.
>
> (p. 7)

Hence, a *material, moral and social revolution* which is allegedly causing a profound sense of insecurity, makes a brief appearance as the causal factor. However, of course, this cannot last. It cannot last, simply because, if this is true at all, then it has to be true for everybody, and as the discourse indicates only 2 per cent of children at risk appear in court; hence the Report argues that 'these major changes in the cultural background may well have replaced the disturbances of war as factors which contribute in themselves to instability within the family' (p. 8), but nevertheless, it is those families which 'Have themselves failed to achieve a stable and satisfactory family life that will be the most vulnerable' (p. 8).

What is being constructed here is ultimately two kinds of family: 'the problem family' and the family 'with a problem'. The services in the community should exist to discover, and provide services for, families with a problem. Hence there must be

> Some centre or body to which parents and others know they can turn for assistance – some door on which they can knock, knowing that their knock will be answered by people with the knowledge and capacity, and with the willingness to help them.
>
> (p. 9)

It could be argued that the above amounts to a virtual denial of class (and gender), certainly of their antagonisms. Unless of course Ingleby is complaining that the power relationships between classes and between the sexes have changed for the worse in that they are more antagonistic, but this is not the connotation here. Also there is no causal connection suggested between class and delinquency. The alleged social and material revolution of the preceding 50 years has, according to the discourse, led to a great deal of uncertainty and anxiety – it is almost as if people no longer know their place – the report even expresses surprise that there is not *more delinquency* – and what prevents it in the majority of cases is the stable functioning family. It hardly seems necessary to add that what therefore produces delinquency in the minority of cases is the lack of such a family.

All of this seems to have implications for the analysis of the Ingleby report advanced by Pitts (1988) who was quoted earlier in this chapter as suggesting that 'the issue of social class is always bubbling just beneath the surface.... The Ingleby Committee... established in 1956 rediscovered this class connection' (p. 2).

It seems therefore that on this occasion Frost and Stein (1989) are much more accurate when they suggest that

> The Report made the link between delinquency and family neglect. The disturbed family came to be seen as the key to both deprivation and depravation. The conflation of these two concepts is the key to understanding the eventual passage of the Children and Young Persons Act 1969.
>
> (p. 36)

However, it is important to remember that the foundations for this conflation were laid in the discourse of the Home Office Children's Branch, 20 years before Ingleby.

Further 'impossibilities' – prediction and prevention

The first chapter of the Ingleby Report concludes with the call for adequate and well coordinated community services with clear and appropriate powers which can properly perform the functions of the ascertainment, diagnosis and treatment of delinquency. Only when this fails or is unlikely to succeed will it be necessary, according to the report, to consider legal sanctions. Hence the closing sentence explains that 'it is for this reason that we have considered the operation of the community services before turning to enquire into the jurisdiction, procedure and powers of the juvenile courts' (p. 9).

The logic of the chapter is crudely instrumental. Essentially it amounts to having 'proper' services in the right place at the right time. Since prevention is the aim this inevitably means that the

> People working in these services, whether they are statutory or voluntary, must have the opportunity to recognise the signs of incipient breakdown in families. Medical practitioners, ministers of religion, teachers, social workers and others must know what they are looking for and how to recognise the danger signals.
>
> (p. 8)

The Report continues by insisting that

> it is important, for instance, to recognise both the obviously inadequate or sub-standard family, and the much less obvious family in which there is a maladjustment of personal relationships; both the classical 'problem family' and what might be called the 'family with a problem'.
>
> (pp. 8–9)

The distinction made by the Report between the two types of family is that in the case of the 'problem family' the 'standards of behaviour and morals will sometimes be as deplorable as the material conditions, but the personal relationships may remain good and helpful to the children.' While on the other hand the 'family with a problem' is one in which 'though outwardly all seems as it should be, the disturbances in the family relationships may be a real danger to them' (p. 9).

The Report adds that it is important that both 'kinds of problem should be discovered early, before things have got too far to be remedied'. In what might in the circumstances be fairly described as an understatement the Report adds, 'it must be recognised that the discovery of these more subtle problems is a very difficult matter' (p. 9).

Chapter 1 of the Ingleby Report clearly privileges the discourse of treatment and prevention, through early identification, over that of judicial procedure. The latter is in the discourse residualised as a last resort to be used only when all else has failed or is clearly failing. There is very little recognition of class, if that means that there is some level of macroeconomic causality seen at the root of delinquency. Deprivation is recognised, but not in 'class terms'. The central focus is instead upon the 'problem family' and the 'family with a problem'. It is the early identification of such families, by everybody from the schoolteacher to the vicar to the social worker to 'others', and their subsequent treatment which is the key. The discourse is able to acknowledge briefly that this is not easy. However, this does not prevent it from taking this crudely instrumental and curative 'scientific' logic several steps further in chapter 7 of the Report, which considers the question of whether local authorities should be given new powers in order to prevent or forestall the suffering of children through neglect and cruelty in their own home.

Ingleby and the problem of cruelty and neglect

Nigel Parton (1985) dismisses the Ingleby Report by suggesting that

> While the remit of the Ingleby Report was to make recommendations on the working of the law in relation to juveniles in trouble, it was also asked to consider 'the prevention of cruelty to, and exposure to moral and physical danger of juveniles', but this was secondary and became consumed by the other concerns so that it virtually disappeared.
>
> (p. 45)

In support of this, Parton simply offers a quote from a secondary source which indicates that in

> dealing with the general issue of the circumstances in which the state may properly intervene in proceedings for child neglect,

the committee states that 'difficulty has not arisen for several years over the reasonable requirements for nutrition, housing, clothing and schooling...' by 1960, then our society had become blind to potential conflicts between family autonomy and child protection.

(Eckelaar *et al.* undated: 76, quoted in Parton 1985: 45)

Nigel Parton continues by proposing that 'in effect the newly emerging social welfare model, with its prime concern on the relationship between neglect and delinquency saw no clash of interests, between the state and different family members' (p. 45). There are several problems with this analysis. In the first place it homogenises the question of neglect with that of cruelty. Hence, in relation to Ingleby on the question of cruelty, which forms chapter 10 of the Ingleby Report, Parton quotes an authority who cites Ingleby on the question of neglect, which is the subject of chapter 2 of Ingleby. Neither is it clear that the Ingleby Report ignores either of these questions, since recommendations are made on both, though it is true that more recommendations are made on other issues.

Familialism, neglect and delinquency

Familialism looms very large in the Ingleby Report, and this is again illustrated in the introductory paragraph of chapter 2 which asserts that 'it is now so widely accepted as to be a commonplace that the problem of the neglected as of the delinquent child is more often than not the problem of the family' (p. 10).

The Report considers the various 'community services' available. It points out that while it is the duty of local authorities under section 1 of the 1948 Act to take children into their care where it appears necessary, it is also subject to subsection (3) which requires the local authority, where this appears consistent with the child's welfare, to ensure that his care is taken over by his parent or guardian, or by a relative or friend.

Prevention, prediction/detection and treatment

The Report recommends that

> There should be a general duty laid upon local authorities to prevent or forestall the suffering of children through neglect in their own homes and local authorities should have the power to do preventive

case-work and to provide material needs that cannot be met from other sources; these powers should be vested generally in the local authority.

(p. 154)

The committee identifies three stages which must be distinguished from each other if prevention and treatment is to be effective. These are

(a) the detection of families at risk;
(b) the investigation and diagnosis of the particular problem;
(c) treatment: the provision of facilities and services to meet the families' needs and to reduce the stresses and dangers that they face.

(p. 17)

The Committee suggests that there is confusion about these different stages and their relative importance. Hence the next six paragraphs of the Report are devoted to outlining these stages. Arrangements for the detection of families at risk, says the committee, 'extend over the widest possible front' (p. 17), and this appears also in the summary of recommendations on page 154 of the Report. The following personnel are recruited to this endeavour:

Neighbours, teachers, medical practitioners, ministers of religion, health visitors, district nurses, education welfare officers, probation officers, child care officers, housing officers, officers of the National Assistance Board may all spot incipient signs of trouble.

(p. 17)

After having spotted 'incipient signs of trouble' one may then move to stage two which concerns investigation and diagnosis. The Committee reports that this issue is

one which many of our witnesses seemed to overlook; they tended to confuse it with detection and treatment. We think it most important that there should be early reference of cases to a unit within the local authority that can give skilled and objective diagnosis.

(p. 18)

Of the third stage, that of treatment, the Report says only that it should remain in the hands of existing agencies though it recognises 'the very valuable work performed by many of the voluntary organisations', and therefore hopes that the local authorities will 'make full use of their powers to make contributions to voluntary bodies engaged in this field' (p. 19).

The Committee also recommends that 'there should be a statutory obligation on all local authorities to submit for ministerial approval schemes for the prevention of suffering of children through neglect in their own homes' (p. 154).

The recommendations in relation to neglect and cruelty

In relation to the question of neglect the Committee makes four recommendations in all. Three of them have been cited above. The fourth urges 'the importance of further study by the Government and local interests concerned of the re-organisation of the various services concerned with the family' (p. 154).

In relation to the question of cruelty, the Report makes further four recommendations. Their first recommendation is that the law should be amended so as to include 'mental suffering' in the definition of cruelty in section 1 of the 1933 Act.

The second permits any department or section of a local authority to instigate proceedings against parents for cruelty and neglect. The reason for this change is because of the development of casework techniques. As a result of them the committee was told that 'there was now less objection to the same department of the local authority prosecuting the parents of the child and caring for the child' (p. 152). Apparently the power was placed originally in the hands exclusively of the education department in order to 'avoid putting the children's committee in the position of prosecutor, as that might make it more difficult for them, in dealing with the child, to secure the parents' cooperation' (p. 152). Clearly the effect of this recommendation is to shift the responsibility for prosecution further towards the children's committee, which of course was ultimately to be integrated into the social services department. Hence, this is an event of significance.

The third recommendation simply brings the fines for cruelty or neglect in line with inflation and the level of other fines.

The fourth recommendation concerns the fact that while the power to imprison in cases of child cruelty and neglect should be retained, nevertheless: 'courts should, in applying the law, make full use of the facilities available for the rehabilitation of the family through residential training or skilled social help' (p. 165). This again illustrates the commitment to treatment over punishment, though it should also be recognised that the power to punish through fines and imprisonment is retained.

The Ingleby Report demands early detection, diagnosis and the treatment of neglect, cruelty and delinquency. It has a crudely instrumental, and very optimistic, view of the efficacy of social casework. It places a statutory responsibility on the local authority to prevent neglect, cruelty and all manner of family difficulty. 'Incipient signs of trouble' must be 'spotted' and acted upon in a three-stage coordinated manner involving detection, diagnosis and treatment. The arrangements for such coordination must be submitted by the local authorities to the Government for approval. Where such preventive work breaks down or where neglect or cruelty is, by the time of referral, so serious as to warrant prosecution, the way is clear for the children's committee to prosecute. In other words, social workers must stop it before it starts, and when they can't or haven't, they must prosecute while also as a first priority 'keeping the family together'.

Decriminalisation and the discourse of treatment

It is clear, from the analysis of the discourse so far, that the Ingleby Report is a discourse of treatment, in the form of prevention, over that of punishment. Essentially it advocates prevention via 'adequate and well co-ordinated community services with clear and appropriate powers'. Only when this fails or is 'clearly unlikely to succeed' will it be necessary to 'fall back on legal sanctions' (p. 9). Nevertheless it does not go so far as to attempt to replace the juvenile court. However, it does move matters explicitly and consciously in such a direction. This is very clear from its recommendation on the subject, which is that the 'juvenile court should be retained but in its dealings with younger children and children whose primary need is for care or protection it should move further away from the conception of criminal jurisdiction' (p. 154).

Since the committee also advocates the raising of the age of criminal responsibility to 12 years, with the possibility of its becoming 13 or 14 at some future date (p. 154), the effect of this recommendation was that any child below that age committing an offence would not be tried for that offence. If they came before the juvenile court at all they would do so as being 'in need of protection and discipline' which was a new procedure that the Committee advocated. The definition of such a person is laid down as follows:

> a person who is in need of protection or discipline is a child who
>
>> (i) is exposed to physical, mental or moral danger; or
>> (ii) is out of control;
>
> and who in any such case, needs care, protection, treatment, control or discipline which is likely to be rejected or unobtainable except by order of a court; or
>
>> (iii) while under the age of twelve years, acts in a manner which would render a person over that age liable to be found guilty of an offence.
>
> (p. 33)

The abolition of the juvenile court

The Report dwells for several paragraphs on the question of the replacement of the juvenile court with a 'non-judicial or quasi-judicial' tribunal, and it says that while it does not agree that the question of the stigma of a court appearance would be avoided by a non-judicial tribunal, since such a tribunal would itself entail such a stigma, the Report nevertheless states that it has

> Some sympathy with the other points made by those who favour a non-judicial tribunal.... A child may be charged with an offence which is not in itself particularly serious, but investigation of which uncovers some serious disturbance in the child or the family situation which requires a great deal of attention. But if the offence is not proved, appropriate action in the interests of the child may not be possible without the institution of new proceedings on a different basis.
>
> (p. 28)

However, for all the disadvantages in judicial proceedings that the Committee members can see, they ultimately conclude that

> One of the difficulties that has impressed us most in considering the suggested alternatives to juvenile courts is that the treatment arranged, or other measures taken, by a non judicial tribunal would depend for their effectiveness ... on the co-operation of the parents

and the child. If... the parents or the child ceased to cooperate, the only remedy would be to bring the case before a court.... We think that the duplication and protraction of proceedings in this way would be undesirable.

(p. 29)

The Ingleby Report, then, was of significance in terms of its contribution to the discourse of treatment over punishment, and while it stopped short of stepping outside judicial procedure altogether, it nevertheless represented a further significant increment of the treatment/welfare discourse.

It remains to compare and contrast Ingleby with the later White Papers *The Child, the Family and the Young Offender* and *Children in Trouble*, both of which were products of a Labour government and each of which formed the basis of the legislation which that government planned.

THE CHILD, THE FAMILY AND THE YOUNG OFFENDER

This is a much thinner document than the Ingleby Report. It contains 13 pages, whereas the Ingleby Report contains 179 pages. The White Paper opens by recalling the Queen's Speech at the opening of the then parliament which indicated that the Government would be concerned to make more effective the means of sustaining the family and of preventing and treating delinquency.

Paragraph 4 delivers the by now familiar promise. It is worth recalling in full because of course it had, in essence, been the position of the Home Office Children's Branch since 1927. It suggests that 'a high proportion of adult criminals have been juvenile delinquents, so that every advance in dealing with the young offender helps also in the attack on adult crime' (p. 3). This is followed immediately by another very familiar theme; the reader is informed that

> The causes of delinquency are complex, and too little is known about them with certainty. It is at least clear that much delinquency – and indeed many other social problems – can be traced back to inadequacy or breakdown in the family. The right place to begin, therefore, is with the family.

(p. 3)

Hence what is clear is that the combination of familialism and the promising of a reduction in both adult and juvenile crime is clearly in operation from the beginning of the document, and in this sense at least the White Paper represents no significant break from past official discourse on the subject.

Decriminalisation and the boundaries of childhood

The first recommendation of the White Paper is that

> Children and young persons under the age of 21 should be regarded as falling into two categories; those under the age of 16, and those between the ages of 16 and 21 .... Sixteen will soon be the upper age for compulsory education. It marks a significant stage in the lives of many young people. It is the age at which they begin to earn, at which they may leave home, at which they may marry. The same consideration has led to the conclusion that this should also be the upper age for the special preventive measures which are applied by law to those children who are in need of care, protection or control and the age after which young persons should in general become subject to the sanctions of the ordinary criminal law.
>
> (p. 5)

The White Paper then moves to consider arrangements for young people under 16. It provides four reasons why it believes these arrangements should be radically changed. They concern the stigma of criminality, and the fact that in the majority of cases brought before the courts the facts of the case are not in dispute. The problem is therefore a question of determining the best treatment, and not the appropriate punishment. The fact that the present arrangements do not provide the best means for getting parents to assume more responsibility for their children's behaviour, and the fact that decisions are made in the form of a court order, which they say allows insufficient flexibility in developing the child's treatment according to his response and changing need (p. 5), are also cited.

Hence, the White Paper proposes that such young people be placed outside the jurisdiction of the juvenile court and the local authority, through its children's committee, is empowered to 'appoint local family councils to deal with each case as far as possible in consultation with the parents' (p. 5).

So far this looks like a relatively clear case of decriminalisation – at least in the case of those under 16. However, in abolishing one court the White Paper promptly suggested establishing two others. The first is the family court. The White Paper suggests that 'where the facts were disputed or agreement could not be reached the case would have to be referred to the family court' (pp. 5–6). In other words the proceedings are still underpinned by a background judicial process since a child below the age of 16 years would have had to plead guilty to avoid criminal proceedings, and a not guilty plea would land her or him in court, albeit a family court.

The second court that the White Paper proposed establishing was the Young Offenders Court. This proposal is contained in paragraph 29 of the White Paper which informs a reader that

> At present offenders under 17 are dealt with in juvenile courts, and offenders between the ages of 17 and 21 are dealt with in the ordinary courts. The special courts, sitting as young offenders' courts, would exercise criminal jurisdiction over offences alleged to have been committed by persons between the ages 16 and 21.
>
> (p. 10)

The White Paper says of its own proposals that they have two main purposes, and they are

> To take children and young persons under the age of 16 as far as possible outside the ambit of the criminal law and the courts, and to make, if possible with the agreement of their parents and guardians, such arrangements for their welfare as are appropriate. The second is to divorce the arrangements for the trial and treatment of young persons in the 16 to 21 age group as far as possible from the ordinary criminal courts and from the penal system as it applies to adults.
>
> (p. 12)

A distinction of degree

It is important to recognise that the distinction between the Ingleby Report and *The Child, the Family and the Young Offender* is a distinction of degree and not one of direction. The latter does not represent a radical break from the former. There is of course a difference, but that difference is essentially accomplished by the White Paper taking the discourse of treatment/prevention one incremental step further. Not so far, however (and this is notwithstanding the no doubt noisy and powerful opposition to the proposals from various interest groups) as to guarantee a final triumph of the discourse of treatment over that of punishment. Indeed the Law, the court, albeit the family court, lurks in the background. It will 'determine' questions of 'the facts' when they are in dispute, that is, it will still determine guilt or innocence. For matters to be dealt with by the family panel, guilt would have to be admitted. While all of this represents a more technical welfarist solution, and therefore a rather less judicial one, it does not amount to decriminalisation. Indeed, in exchange for one court we get two – albeit both with a welfare principle at their centre. It is as if treatment and punishment cannot manage without each other; without welfare, punishment would be stripped bare, and, without justice, welfare would stand naked.

Ford (1975) is a particularly interesting commentator on this period. He was, in fact, a member of the Ingleby Committee, a magistrate and one-time Chairman of the London County Council Children's Committee. His book is a 'Study of The Children and Young Persons Act 1969'. He is a supporter of the Act. In relation to Family Councils he suggests that

> Many times a court is faced with parents who want a child to plead guilty to an offence, so that an action can be concluded with dispatch. If this can happen in a court setting...how much greater is the danger in the context of a family council?
>
> (p. 16)

He also objects on the basis that

> The family council...would not be subject to scrutiny.... In the end I came down *marginally*, against the idea of a family council because I felt that the rights of the child and the parents were better safeguarded by some form of judicial procedure in the first instance.... On that basis, and it was *agonisingly marginal, I* came to the conclusion that the juvenile court should survive.
>
> (pp. 16–17, my emphasis)

What is interesting here is the fact that, for one member at least of the Ingleby Committee, the decision to be taken in relation to the abolition of the juvenile court was agonisingly marginal, precisely because he could not sanction a significant increase in bureaucratic power without a judicial referee. Of course it is also clear from his strong support of the 1969 Act that he cannot either sanction judicial power outside the context of the presence of welfare acting as a referee. This further reinforces the idea that the distinction between Ingleby and *The Child, the Family and the Young Offender* was itself in an important sense marginal; certainly it gives no credence to the view that it represented a radical break from past practice.

In the event, because of opposition from interest groups which stood to lose power and influence, the Government had to compromise. The fruit of that compromise was the White Paper entitled *Children in Trouble*, and it was this that was to form the basis of the 1969 Act. It is to an analysis of the discourse of this White Paper that this chapter now turns.

CHILDREN IN TROUBLE – A DISCOURSE OF COMPROMISE

Immediately following five introductory paragraphs, the White Paper, under the heading 'General', states its position in relation to juvenile delinquency. The opening paragraph of these observations is particularly interesting, and is worth analysing in detail. The first five sentences inform the reader that juvenile delinquency

> has no single cause, manifestation, or cure. Its origins, and the range it covers is equally wide. At some points it merges almost imperceptibly with behaviour which does not contravene the law. A child's behaviour is influenced by genetic, emotional and intellectual factors, his maturity, and his family, school, neighbourhood and wider social setting. It is probably a minority of children who grow up without ever misbehaving in ways which may be contrary to the law. Frequently such behaviour is no more than an incident in the pattern of a child's normal development.
>
> (pp. 3–4)

Two of the sentences, the first and third, are statements about the causes of and influences upon juvenile behaviour. In the case of sentence number one, the subject is juvenile delinquency, which is said to have no single cause, manifestation or cure. The subject of sentence number three is a child's behaviour, that is, general behaviour, inclusive of delinquent behaviour, which is influenced by three general factors – the genetic, the emotional and the intellectual – and five specific factors: his maturity, his family, school, neighbourhood and his wider social setting. These two sentences are neutral in relation to the importance or significance of juvenile delinquency.

The other three sentences, however, are not neutral about the importance of juvenile delinquency. Sentences two, four and five seem to minimise the issue. Sentence two suggests that there are some points at which delinquent behaviour is indistinguishable from non-delinquent behaviour since it merges imperceptibly with it. Sentence four seems to suggest that the majority of children are delinquent, since it is probably a minority who grow up without ever misbehaving. Sentence five appears to suggest to a reader that the delinquent behaviour is often quite normal, since it is frequently no more than an incident in the pattern of normal development.

Given all this, a reader may be forgiven for wondering why a White Paper has been produced at all, since apparently we often don't know whether young people are being delinquent or not, and anyway, at some time or another most of them are, and furthermore, it's normal. However, a reader is not permitted such potential illusions for long, for the sixth sentence begins with an all-important 'But' and continues by suggesting that

> Sometimes it is a response to unsatisfactory social circumstances, a result of boredom in and out of school, an indication of maladjustment or immaturity, or a symptom of a deviant, damaged or abnormal personality. Early recognition and full assessment are particularly important in these more serious cases.
>
> (p. 4)

Having suggested that at least sometimes delinquency is far from normal, the discourse moves to the social consequences of juvenile delinquency, which range from minor nuisance to considerable damage and suffering for the community. It continues by informing a reader that 'an important object of the criminal law is to protect society against such consequences, but the community also recognises the importance of caring for those who are too young to protect themselves' (p. 4).

The Law and the community in harmony

This distinction between a caring/suffering/warm/passive community, and a colder/active/protective 'law'/Law is then pressed into further service by the discourse since it immediately suggests that

> Over recent years these two quite distinct grounds for action by society have been moving steadily closer together. It has become increasingly clear that social control of harmful behaviour by the young, and social measures to help and protect the young, are not distinct and separate processes. The aims of protecting society from juvenile delinquency, and of helping children in trouble to grow up into more mature and law-abiding persons, are complementary and not contradictory.
>
> (p. 4)

It could also be suggested that this discursive device of radically dichotomising the law and the community, only to bring them together again in a virtuous reunion, represents an attempt to produce a compromise between the various interest groups that had fallen out over the previous White Paper. The legal profession must be reassigned their proper place, the Law must protect society, while the caring profession must also have its due, and the community must care, no doubt with the able assistance of those allegedly skilled in these matters. Both are of equal value, at least in discursive terms, and at least so far.

The White Paper explicitly acknowledges that there was some negative response to its predecessor *The Child, the Family and the Young Offender*. It reports that there were many comments that young people could better be kept out of courts on

> an informal basis by social workers, rather than through family councils; and that the basic choice over the procedure to be adopted in each individual case should therefore lie between, on the one hand, court proceedings and, on the other, the provision of help and guidance on an entirely voluntary basis.
>
> (p. 5)

The White Paper then offers the compromise solution in which

> The procedure for children under 10 will remain as at present; there will be new provisions for those aged 10 and under 14, which will be added to those relating to children under 10, and new provisions also for those over 14 and under 17 which will be added to those relating to the younger age groups. The procedure for offenders aged 10 and under 14 will narrow down the circumstances

in which court proceedings are now possible. It represents a half way stage between care, protection or control proceedings and prosecution.

(p. 5)

Sentenced to treatment

In these proposals, of course, the juvenile court was retained, and for 10- to 14-year-old children the committing of an offence ceased to be, in itself, sufficient grounds for bringing them to court. Where it was necessary to bring a child of this age before a court, it became also necessary to establish that the offender was 'not receiving such care, protection or guidance as a good parent may reasonably be expected to give, or is beyond control' (p. 6). The purpose of this was, of course, to reduce the number of such children appearing in court, via the insertion of the 'trip wire' outlined earlier (see Ford 1975: 24). In addition to this, it also changed the basis of such court appearances. The powers of the juvenile court in relation to this age group were 'committal to care of local authority, Supervision with or without intermediate treatment, Hospital or guardianship order under the Mental Health Act, Binding over parents' (p. 18).

It can be seen that none of these 'disposals' involve, at a formal/ technical level a 'punitive' response, since of course the only ground for the child's being before the court is the question of care and control. Therefore, it could be argued that this represented a decriminalisation. However, whether the finer points of this technicality were clear to either the children concerned, or their parents, is perhaps another matter. After all, you could still get 'put away', even if being *put away* meant that you were in the care of the local authority, in a local children's home, and you were there not because you were 'guilty' but because you were 'in need of care and control'.

In the case of 16- and 17-year-olds, there was the attempt to keep as many as possible out of the juvenile court, and the attempt, where that had failed, to restrict the use of the more obviously punitive responses, that is, attendance centres, detention, approved school and borstals.

This was to be achieved by a dual strategy. In the case of the attendance centre and the detention centre the White Paper announces that 'provision will be made for new forms of intermediate treatment, for use in conjunction with supervision, to be developed by local authorities. These will in due course replace junior attendance centres, and junior detention centres' (p. 17). In relation to approved school and borstal training, the White Paper envisages that

> Children and young persons requiring continuing treatment away from home will be placed in the care of local authorities. The separate approved school order will cease to exist, and borstal for those over 17 will in due course be replaced.
>
> (p. 17)

This of course represents a restriction on the number of punitive disposals available to the court. In the event, not all of the 'decriminalisation' proposals were implemented. The Conservative government coming to power in June 1970 announced its intention to shelve them. Had the White Paper's proposals been fully implemented, criminal proceedings would have been possible only for those between 14 and 17 years of age. The only *punitive* disposal that the White Paper envisaged in such proceedings, apart from an absolute or conditional discharge, was a fine of up to £50, and the payment of damages or compensation. Detention centres and attendance centres were to remain available until such times as intermediate treatment became available.

Intermediate treatment

As its name implies, this form of treatment was intermediate between a child or young person's home and a residential facility. Appendix C of the White Paper says of intermediate treatment that

> Where possible a child or young person under supervision should be treated as a member of his local community and in association with others of his own age, and treatment of this kind should not be restricted to groups of delinquents alone. It is important therefore to make the best co-operative use of all available local resources and services, both statutory and voluntary ... the basic responsibility for their provision should be local rather than central.
>
> (p. 22)

In relation to all of the above it is important to recognise that there is an important level at which justice and welfare are parasitic upon each other. They are parasitic upon each other because they mark out for each other the boundaries of the subject. The struggle between the two poles of this discursive phenomenon – treatment/administrative responses and punishment/judicial responses – is not at all about abolishing these discursive boundaries. The question at issue is about the distribution of power and influence within these parameters, and only very rarely does either side of the debate raise the question of the parameters themselves. Indeed it often seems to be the case that in the heat and smoke of their battle the very existence of the parameters is obscured from view.

This chapter has considered the official discourse in relation to both the 1963 and the 1969 Children and Young Persons Act. The major innovations in both of them related to the question of juvenile delinquency. However, it remains important to remember that care proceedings for child abuse – inclusive of course of sexual abuse, emotional abuse and neglect – took place until November 1991 under the (subsequently amended) 1969 Act, as did the provision relating to a Place of Safety, though there was also a (slightly different) provision for the latter available under the 1933 Act. The usual provision under which care proceedings took place in relation to child abuse was under section 1(a) of the 1969 Act which permits such proceedings if 'His (or her) proper development is being avoidably prevented or neglected or his (or her) health is being avoidably impaired or neglected or he/she is being ill-treated'. In the light of this, it does not seem entirely accurate to suggest that

> Under the 1969 Children and Young Persons Act children in trouble with the law were treated in virtually the same way as children who were not offenders. In the process of conceptualising and treating all problems to do with children as being essentially the same, any reference to children as victims was lost. It is almost as if it was assumed that a conflict of interests between child, parents and the state had disappeared and the nineteenth-century problems of cruelty and neglect had been virtually abolished.
>
> (Parton 1985: 45)

While there is quite clearly some truth in the idea that an uncritical adherence to a naive familialism and a similarly naive overconfidence in the ability to predict problems and prevent them will no doubt obscure from view the potential for the oppression of both women and children in a 'normal' family, it can hardly be said that the problems of cruelty and neglect had virtually been abolished.

Instead, it would be more appropriate and accurate to recognise the continuity, but to see that continuity as the incremental and evolutionary emergence of the discourse of treatment against punishment. This is not to say, of course, that this was not a politically contested phenomenon, indeed at the two poles of the discourse stood those with a vested interest and therefore with the most to gain from their own preferred outcome, that is, the legal expert and the non-legal administrative expert. The late 1960s represented the (short-lived) high-water mark of the struggle of treatment to supplant punishment. However, neither can ever fully defeat the other since, as has been suggested earlier, they are parasitic upon each other.

Hence in offering a critique of either pole of this discursive struggle one must take great care, via criticising one, not to appear to uphold the other, since this would only breathe further life into their struggle and as a result further obscure the boundaries of each discourse which, in turn, would further serve to keep the delinquents and their caretakers/households and families for ever entangled within them – as prisoners of justice, or as prisoners of treatment. It is also important to remember, of course, that merely because the contest is motivated, it does not follow that there is no truth, or indeed altruism, on either side of it.

Such a critique in recognising continuity would also need to avoid seeing this continuity as a 'steady march of progress'. Neither this, nor a theory which sees only, or mainly, radical breaks occurring solely because of class struggle or moral panic, etc. will do. It is a question of recognising the continuity as a discursive phenomenon, a phenomenon which is not immune from taking important twists or turns as a result of class struggle or moral panic, etc. but which will nevertheless survive and may even mobilise such struggle or panic. This is, of course, barring such a fundamental political transformation as to render no longer operable the power relations which sustain both poles of the struggle.

Chapter 7

Moral panic and Maria Colwell

The previous chapter, in considering the period in British childcare legislation which is generally taken to represent the triumph of the discourse of treatment over punishment, argued that while the period represented the 'high-water mark' of the discourse of treatment, it was nevertheless not accurate to see this as the triumph of treatment. The chapter confronted in particular the arguments of Pitts (1988) and also Frost and Stein (1989) and suggested that in setting too much store by the reforming zeal of a Labour government they overstated the treatment side of the dichotomy and thus underestimated the extent to which it is still firmly underpinned by the discourse of punishment. The chapter argued that the two discourses are in an important sense parasitic upon each other, while it nevertheless remains true that, in particular periods, one end of the dichotomy may appear in sharper relief than the other.

An essential fault line of the position is that it overlooks the continuity of the British state as a source and bearer for such discourses and ideologies and it therefore falls prey to placing too great an emphasis on sudden breaks with past law, policy and practice, purely and only explicable by such concepts as a Labour government reflecting class struggle or the reactionary intentions of a Conservative government, or moral panic.

THE ROLE PLAYED BY MORAL PANIC

The current chapter critically examines this last approach, that is, the question of the role played by moral panic in rendering child (physical) abuse as a matter for urgent attention, and also in the production of the 1975 Children Act. It should be emphasised at the outset that the chapter does not deny the existence of such a panic. It is not my argument that breaks and shifts of emphasis do not happen or even that a part of the explanation for them does not lie in factors in operation at the time of the framing of the legislation. It is rather that such shifts of emphasis, sudden and sharp as they may appear to be, nevertheless have longer-standing ideological and discursive roots.

The continuity of the British State is succinctly illustrated, albeit particularly in relation to the 1945 Labour government, by Addison (1975) when he quotes Richard Crossman as asking

> How much more humane and imaginative our post war reconstruc-
> tion would have proved if government departments had been
> invigorated by an influx of experts with special knowledge, new
> ideas and sympathy for the Government's...policies. But the
> Premier dismissed such suggestions as Left-wing claptrap. Once
> again, as after 1918, the best of the temporary civil servants
> returned to their peacetime occupations and the old establishment
> ruled unchallenged over a bureaucratic empire which had been
> enormously enlarged and dangerously centralised during the war.
>
> (pp. 277–8)

The importance of this lies in the recognition that it is a mistake to simply consider legislative and policy 'shifts in relation to factors out-side the state and its bureaucracy. What is required is consideration of what is taking place both within the state and outside it, and a consider-ation of the interaction of both. Hence the chapter, in attempting this, will first outline the position of Parton (1985) on the question of moral panic in relation to the death of Maria Colwell. It will then examine some of the discourse contained in the *Report of the Committee of Inquiry into the Care and Supervision Provided in Relation to Maria Colwell* (DHSS 1974). It should be acknowledged that the *Report of the Departmental Committee on the Adoption of Children* (Houghton Committee 1972) was also important in framing the legislation in ques-tion, since there is wide agreement that both of these reports were major influences on the construction of the 1975 Act (see, for instance, Fox Harding 1991; Frost and Stein 1989; Parton 1985; Stevenson 1989).

Maria Colwell

It is appropriate to focus this chapter on the specific case of Maria Colwell, since the views of Parton (1985) are influential in the social-work field and they centralise a moral panic about this case as the major determining factor in producing a particular societal response to the issue in question. Considering this case closely establishes and clarifies the fact that the detail of the discourse is still firmly located within the historic discourses of child protection with which this book is engaged. In particular it concerns a specific question within the ideology/discourse of familialism, that is, that of the importance of 'the blood tie' over a social/psychological tie. In other words it concerns centrally the issue of the claims of the biological parent over that of the social/psychological (foster) parent. It concerns what the media of the day termed a 'tug of love', and the dilemma in which a social worker and her agency found themselves in relation to attempting to resolve it. It concerns the tragic death, at the hands of her stepfather, of a young girl.

This question of 'the blood tie' is central in the Maria Colwell case because Maria Colwell died at the hands of her stepfather after being returned to her mother following a long period in the foster care of relatives of her mother. The inquiry report contains a minority report, and the area of disagreement within the committee is precisely on this question, that is, it concerns the wisdom of the decision of East Sussex County Council not to oppose the revocation of the Care Order relating to Maria Colwell, thus returning her to her biological parent, and of course her stepfather. For this reason, particular attention is paid to this aspect of the discourse, in both of the majority and minority reports. Careful attention to the specific discourse contained in the report sheds a different and, in my view, clearer light on the matter in hand. However, it is necessary first to outline the position which is to be criticised.

Moral panic

In 1973 Stanley Cohen argued that

> Societies seem to be subject, every now and then to periods of moral panic. A condition, episode, person or group of persons emerges to become defined as a threat to societal values and interests . . . sometimes the object of the panic is quite novel and at other times it is something that has been in existence long enough but suddenly appears in the limelight.
>
> (Cohen 1973: 9)

Parton (1985) devotes a chapter to the issue of a moral panic in relation to Maria Colwell, and in it 1975 Act is held to be in a major sense a product of the societal reaction to her death. The Act did of course represent a more pessimistic view of the discourse of treatment as against punishment, and as a result the state was markedly more inclined to intervene into 'the family' in order not simply to 'treat' families and children, but also to separate them. The quote below, from a then Director of Social Services, writing in the preface of a guidebook for social workers on childcare law, gives a flavour of the professional reaction at the time to the extent of the shift, when he warns that

> The backlash marked by the Children's Act 1975 displays, one hopes, the limits of the pendulum's swing. Parents voluntarily entrusting their children to the care of local authorities or voluntary agencies must be warned that they risk losing their parental status for no other reason than that their inability to care for them has continued for three years.
>
> (Brill 1976: viii)

Clearly there is in this Act a shift of importance which does require some explanation. In order to offer such an explanation Parton himself leans heavily upon the work of Hall *et al.* (1978). He mobilises and modifies their work in order to locate the social reaction to the death of Maria Colwell within the wider theme of the 'violent society'. He points out that

> Hall *et al.* argue . . . that there has taken place a change in the nature of moral panics in the post war period whereby there has been a 'mapping together' of previously discrete moral panics into a more general panic about the social order and the increasing level of violence throughout society, culminating in 1972–73 with a 'law and order' campaign. It thus is important to see how far the panic about child abuse was related to a more general moral panic at the time, and how far it symbolised a 'more widespread social morass' in British society in the early 1970's.
>
> (Parton 1985: 72)

Parton, in a footnote, distances himself from Hall *et al.* and suggests that 'it is far from apparent that S. Hall *et al.*'s grand theory that moral panics in the early 1970s were part of a wider crisis is valid' (p. 216). Nevertheless this does not prevent him from centralising this as a very important part, if not the central part, of the explanation for the emergence of child (physical) abuse as a major focus of attention.

He suggests this in the first sentence of his section headed 'Conclusions'. It is worth quoting the sentence in full.

> In this chapter I have argued that it was the inquiry into the death of Maria Colwell late in 1973 that was the crucial event in establishing the issue as a major social problem and for providing the catalyst for the rapid emergence of a 'moral panic'. The efforts of the Tunbridge Wells Study Group, Sir Keith Joseph, and the D.H.S.S., while central to this process, were also dependent upon and fed into significant changes in the socio-political climate of the time.
>
> (p. 97)

Nigel Parton grafts child abuse onto a moral panic which, while containing a number of themes, nevertheless converges in the central theme of 'the violent society'. There are a number of problems in doing so and they are outlined below.

On page 82 of Parton (1985), is reproduced, from Chibnall (1977), a 'map' entitled 'The Violent Society: emergence of themes'. In it is depicted the convergence of a 'Criminal violence theme' and a 'Political violence theme', both of which commence in the mid-1960s. It depicts the convergence of, on the one hand, the Moors murders, the Krays, etc. and, on the other hand, student demonstrations, the IRA, the Angry Brigade, violent picketing, etc.: These together produce the theme of the violent society which then coalesces around 'mugging' in 1972–3 and the IRA mainland bombing campaign of 1973. The central question to be faced is the extent to which it is possible to sensibly add to the above child (physical) abuse in 1974 through the Maria Colwell inquiry. In other words, quite independently of the validity of the map itself up until that time, does child abuse fit easily on to the end of it? To place it there seems to raise a number of conceptual questions.

Racism

In the first place it is important to remember the central dimension of an analysis of racism in the work of Hall *et al*. Parton does not refer to this; and while the media may well have presented the case of Maria Colwell as cause for concern, there was not the suggestion that there was a child killer lurking around every corner – but a mugger, or a terrorist bomb in your neighbourhood, or on your transport system, perhaps. There is a suggested randomness about these latter things. They can allegedly happen to any and all of us at any time (even if in fact they don't): but they may be just around the corner, your corner, and this is the fear that such a panic generates, and in a literal sense is. Child abuse, however, happens only to some children, and the fact that it is perpetrated by people who may be characterised as 'monsters' or 'evil', does not mean that the perpetrators are seen in quite the same light as, for instance, terrorists.

In terms of legitimation for a 'law and order' campaign the radical otherness of terrorists or (allegedly black) 'muggers' or even violent pickets is crucial. After all it is a *they* who should be dealt with, and firmly at that. But when it comes to child abuse, even where it is recognised as a minority phenomenon, it nevertheless takes place in a very literal sense at home, in 'the family'. If it is to be 'sorted out' it is *we* who must be sorted out. There is all the difference in the world between going along with strong action against *them* and strong action against us or even me.

This is not a trivial difference. After all, we are considering the split between the public and the private and this is important in understanding why, by the late 1980s, there was public concern when the media became critical of social workers for intervening in 'the family' to too great an extent. The issue was still child abuse, though the focus was on child sexual abuse. It could be suggested that neither the initial criticism for intervening too little nor the later criticism for intervening too much can be properly understood without a focus upon the ideology/discourse of familialism. Both the 'too little' approach, and the 'too much' can be handled when it is placed in this context: for example, too little endeavour to protect the family on the one hand, and too much invasion of its sanctity on the other. In the context of a moral panic the idea of a 'too much intervention' approach becomes mysterious indeed.

Violence against women

A further point needs to be made in relation to this. If there was a moral panic about violence, and it included violence in 'the family', then why was violence against women in their own homes not as important an issue? It is, of course, possible to offer an explanation of this by a consideration of male power but this is not (in 1985) a part of Parton's analysis either.

The identified 'culprit'

There is a further crucial difference and it relates to the identified 'culprit'. When a terrorist plants a bomb, people understandably enough blame the terrorist. When a robbery is committed the thief is held to be responsible. However, Parton himself quotes coverage in *The Times*, and in each of the five headlines he offers on the Maria Colwell inquiry the subject of the headline is social workers: for example, 'Social worker booed at Brighton inquiry'. When the terrorist plant a bomb people do not come to court in order to boo the Special Branch. When a picket appears in court charged with violence, only militant trade unionists are likely to come to court in order to express their displeasure at the local constabulary. People certainly do not boo the police when black youths stand accused of 'mugging'. There is a difference of huge significance between the identified culprit in the case of violence against children as compared with the violence of terrorists, muggers etc. Once this central difference is grasped it is no longer possible to see media concern about child (physical) abuse, however seemingly unfair and apparently irrational, as simply part and parcel of a more general moral panic about 'a violent society'.

The discursive roots of the 'moral panic'

The difference in the identified culprit in these cases can of course be explained with reference to the continuity of the discourses and ideologies in British childcare legislation with which this book is concerned. It is quite a simple difference; perhaps its very simplicity partly explains why it is so often overlooked. It is that the discourses finding their way into British childcare legislation are different from those which apply to the police. Police people would, through their federation, perhaps have something to say, along no doubt with the rest of us, if they had a statutory responsibility to prevent crime, to discover crime, to intervene before a crime is committed in order to prevent it, and where a crime is committed to then make endeavours where possible to keep 'the (criminal) family' together.

If by an admittedly wild stretch of the imagination this could be envisaged, it would require very little, if any, further imagination to realise that, given this exceptionally tall order, they would at times, quite simply, get it wrong. One would then require no further imagination at all to realise that there would be cases in which public inquiries were held to establish what went wrong, since in relation to his or her statutory duties a police person had 'got it wrong'. If there was a great deal of media coverage, and the particular area in which the mistake had been made was a highly emotive one, then one might also be able to imagine some people attending the public inquiry and booing the hapless and, no doubt, bewildered constable.

The problem of the social-work task in itself

The point of the earlier imagining is, of course, to illustrate that social workers are charged with statutory responsibilities which the police are not. It is this which is the fully rational core of the differential treatment of, for instance, Special Branch or other anti-terrorist police squads, when it comes to terrorist bombers, etc., compared with social workers in child abuse cases. It is also why the two things need to be kept firmly separate. To lump them together risks missing a very important point, and it is simply this: however unfair and apparently irrational the media coverage may be, the sad fact is that there is a real question to be asked about what went wrong.

It is not, in my view, enough to say 'don't panic'. Quite apart from anything else it is in the nature of panics that this sort of advice is rarely taken. It is not a total solution either to keep putting forward candidates for aids in carrying out these onerous statutory duties: for example, better methods of prediction, or more inter-agency cooperation. These may be helpful, or not, depending upon that which is suggested. The point of following the discourses of the legislation which produced both the task, and those expected to carry it out, that is, LA social workers, is to critically examine the emergence of the task itself. Perhaps too much is being asked of too few? Perhaps the order is too tall, and too contradictory, and no doubt at times nearly impossible. Certainly absolutely impossible if those charged with carrying out the task are expected to get it right every time. The double difficulty of this is that when it is 'got wrong' the results are often tragic, both for the child and for the social worker.

In fairness to Nigel Parton is should be pointed out that by 1990 he had distanced himself from some aspects of his earlier work. However, he does not distance himself from that part of his analysis which is criticised earlier. In fact he reasserts its importance. In order to illustrate this adequately, it is fair to quote him on his recantation of some aspects of this work, and also on his reassertion of the importance of the concept of moral panic. He recants on some of his analysis, under the heading 'The failure to recognise the child in child abuse' by indicating that

> It was evident from the outset that *The Politics of Child Abuse* was inadequate in a least three areas; its failure to address sexual abuse; its difficulties in taking into account the dimension of gender; and its ambiguous messages for the practitioner.
>
> (Parton 1991: 10)

He adds that there was a fundamental problem in the analysis itself and suggests that this was related to an uncritical adoption of the sociology of deviance. He suggests that a later critique of such theories 'therefore informed and skewed the analysis developed in *The Politics of Child Abuse*' (p. 10).

However, the absences of the issues he outlines do not alone account for the inadequacy of the book since, if he had recognised the 'category mistake' involved in grafting child abuse onto a moral panic about a 'violent society', this might well have pushed him to consider the emergence of the issue over a longer period. When one reads the various documents which form much of the raw material of this book, their uncritical approach to gender and 'the family', and their inherent ethnocentricity are, in fact, hard to miss.

In the light of all the above it should clearly be acknowledged that the work of Nigel Parton was pioneering in the sense that it raised very important questions for serious discussion. Also the focus in this chapter has been in relation to his centralising the emergence of the problem of child (physical) abuse in the mid-1970s within the context of moral panic. This is, of course, not all that he has to say on the subject. He usefully outlines the way in which particular forms of research were influential in producing a shift of emphasis. He suggests, for instance, that prior to 1968 there was still

> A significant element of the control culture that located the problem on the 'border-line between medicine and the law'. But increasingly after 1969, under the influence of the NSPCC Battered Child Research Unit the problem was conceptualised squarely in terms of a medical and social welfare problem.
>
> (Parton 1985: 97)

It is important to consider the activities of influential research units. However, the earlier implies that the role of the law was becoming less important by 1968. But of course it is precisely through the law that the Maria Colwell case was a case at all. The law does not forget, even where we forget it, and furthermore it already contains medical and social welfare discourses – it provides the context for and the boundaries of the very kinds of shifts of emphasis which Nigel Parton's work is an attempt to explain. It is therefore important to consider the actual discourses contained in the *Report of the Committee of Inquiry into the Care and Supervision Provided in Relation to Maria Colwell*.

REPORT OF THE COMMITTEE OF INQUIRY INTO THE CARE AND SUPERVISION PROVIDED IN RELATION TO MARIA COLWELL

On 17 July 1973, Sir Keith Joseph appointed a Committee of Inquiry into the Care and Supervision Provided in Relation to Maria Colwell. The report was presented to Barbara Castle, the then Secretary of State for Social Services, 9 months later. The report is lengthy; it covers 118 pages. There is not a unanimous view presented by the committee. Ms Olive Stevenson presented her own minority report which forms chapter 5 of the report. The discourse articulates around the issue of the claims of the natural (biological) parent, against the claims of the social/psychological (foster) parent. The question of violence to a child is of course centrally involved.

However, what needs to be kept in mind is the fact that the violence involved in this particular case might not have taken place had the care of Maria not been handed over to her biological mother, and her new partner, which involved removing Maria from foster parents with whom she was apparently very happy. The text of both the majority and the minority report is centrally concerned with the activities of social workers in relation to the claims of a biological parent over that of foster parents.

Prior to moving into the report proper, however, it is important to make some observations in relation to such public inquiries. Hallett (1989) provides an analysis of child abuse inquiries in which she points to the long and continuing tradition of such public inquiries in British social policy. For instance the list provided for the Kimberley Carlile report included 34 such reports. These may range from internal inquiries to external inquiries instigated by the local authority, and to those instituted by the Secretary of State for Social Services. There are differences too in the way such inquiries may go about their task. The proceedings may be adversarial or inquisitorial, and the inquiry may be statutory or non-statutory.

In the case of the Maria Colwell Inquiry the proceedings were adversarial, but not statutory. In other words, because the Inquiry was non-statutory the witnesses appeared voluntarily, and because it was adversarial the truth was established via cross-examination etc. No witnesses requested to attend the Maria Colwell inquiry refused to do so, but the problems that might have arisen were noted, and as a result the power to set up a statutory inquiry was incorporated into the Children Act 1975 in Section 98 (2) (see Hallett 1989: 112). It has been the case since that, in non-statutory inquiries, social workers and doctors have on occasions followed the advice of their trade union, or their medical defence union, and refused to give oral evidence.

It is worth bearing in mind, of course, that since all inquiries are concerned to establish 'the truth', they are all in an important sense therefore 'inquisitorial'. Appearing at such an inquiry would no doubt be a traumatic experience whatever form it took. Clearly there is a difference between a version of events that resides in an individual participant's thoughts, on the one hand, and the translation of the participant's individual thoughts on the matter, in so far as they are elicited, into the official version of events which forms the discourse of the inquiry report on the other. This is true even where the committee does not present a unanimous view.

This cautionary note is included in order to illustrate that it is not the purpose of this section of the chapter to elicit 'the truth' of the matter in hand; it is rather to elicit the 'truth' of the discourse itself. It is concerned with the parameters within which the discourse takes place. It is engaged with the concerns of the discourse itself. Nevertheless, some observations will be made, outside the context of the discourse itself, which refer to the dilemma in which the social workers involved found themselves.

The narrow focus of public inquiries

There is one further cautionary note to be struck. Such inquiries are concerned with the detail of the implementation of law and policy. They are not concerned with issues of resources, let alone issues in any wider context. What is under investigation is a specific event, or specific events, and not a general problem. Hence they will inevitably tend to be individually focused; they will be in the main concerned with what went wrong and with who is to blame. Of course, it may be that such inquiries in their reports step outside of their terms of reference and make general observations, but first they must address the issues raised by their terms of reference. The Maria Colwell Inquiry stayed within its terms of reference except in so far as it made the observation in relation to voluntary participation which is outlined earlier. It is important to bear in mind the narrowness of this focus. For instance, the Department of Transport in the inquiry into the sinking of the Zeebrugge ferry focused all the blame on the individual who failed to close the doors and none of the blame on the management of the company for not having a more fail-safe safety routine, including the installation of warning lights. It did not criticise the government either for not legislating more stringently on the question of safety at sea. This observation is made simply because it is important to recognise the narrowness of the focus of the Inquiry, and therefore of the discourse which I intend to consider.

The report contains five chapters; they are: 1. Introduction; 2. Narrative; 3. Comments; 4. Conclusion; and 5. Minority Report on Events up to 22 November 1971. The introduction is brief. The narrative on the other hand is by far the longest chapter, and it contains 138 paragraphs. For the purposes of this analysis I will first very briefly summarise the essentials of the narrative, only quoting the Report where necessary. However, when I outline some of the comments and conclusions I will, of course, quote the Report and where necessary quote and/or summarise any detail of the narrative to which the comment or conclusion quoted specifically refers. I will also outline areas of disagreement within the committee by a consideration of the minority report of Ms Olive Stevenson.

Narrative

East Sussex Children's Department first became involved with the Colwell Family in January of 1965. They were said to have 'multiple problems'. Mr Colwell died 6 months later. Mrs Colwell then placed Maria, aged then 6 months, with a Mrs and Mr Cooper. Mrs Cooper was Mrs Colwell's sister-in-law. The Coopers had brought up their own children, and they had an adult daughter living with them.

After Mr Colwell's death Mrs Colwell 'went to pieces' (paragraph 14, p. 11 of the Report). Her other four children, all older than Maria, according to an NSPCC report quoted in the same paragraph, 'stopped going to school altogether; Mrs Colwell made no effort to help herself and did not use any of the constructive help offered by myself or other social workers'. Ultimately the four older children were removed on a Place of Safety Order and a Care Order was made on 15 December 1965, in relation to the four children other than Maria. Maria remained for the time being at the Coopers'. This was a voluntary arrangement, and in July 1966 Mrs Colwell removed Maria from the Coopers, which she was thus entitled to do. A week later she placed Maria with a family who were known to the NSPCC, and Maria was removed from them on a Place of Safety Order. On 17 August 1966 Maria was taken into the care of East Sussex County Council. She was placed back with Mrs Cooper, but now this arrangement was statutory and not voluntary. According to the report for Hove Juvenile Court, of 17 November 1971,

> Maria made very good progress with Mr and Mrs Cooper and was much loved by this family. The care she received from them contributed towards her basically stable and happy personality. She regarded foster-parents as 'Mummy and Daddy' though aware of her relationship to them and to her siblings.
>
> (Lees, D., social worker ESCC,
Appendix 3: 119)

What changed the situation, and what was therefore the reason for the court report, was that Mrs Colwell had decided to apply for the revocation of the Care Order. The report argued that while Mrs Colwell between 1967 and 1969 had an unsettled way of life and maintained only irregular contact with the children, having apparently 17 addresses during that period, nevertheless by

> April 1969 at the time of her penultimate move, we became aware of her cohabitation with Mr Kepple as an ongoing relationship. This cohabitation has since been maintained and an apparently stable family relationship now exists. The couple have stated their intention to marry in the near future. Altogether there has been a very considerable improvement in Mrs Colwell's total situation.
>
> (p. 119)

The court report disclosed that, in the previous year, ESCC were making attempts to increase the contact between Maria and her mother with a view of 'building a relationship with them'. While 'such a relationship has grown', the situation was complicated by the 'strong feeling of mutual dislike between the Kepples and the foster parents' and a 'situation akin to a feud has developed' (p. 120). The report suggested that because of this Maria was 'in some confusion over where her loyalties lie' (p. 120). Because of this apparent conflict of loyalties the report suggested that a gradual return of Maria to her mother was 'out of the question' and added that

> It is felt that her future needs would probably best be met if she was with her mother, although this was not an easy or clear-cut decision. With this in mind Maria returned home on trial to her mother on 22 October 1971. She was extremely unhappy about parting with the

Coopers, but calmed down on seeing her mother. Since her return she has run away to some nearby Cooper relatives on one occasion, but again appeared to return happily to her mother when she saw her.

(Appendix 3: 119)

The court report concluded by suggesting that Maria's return to her mother was 'proving successful so far', and that it would therefore be in her best interests for 'the Care Order to be revoked'. However

In view of the difficulties which have already been experienced in this situation, and the strain imposed on Maria by parting from her foster parents, the Court might wish to consider the possibility of making a supervision order.

(Appendix 3: 119)

The court followed the recommendation. Maria died of multiple head injuries at the age of 7, in January 1973. William Kepple was charged with her murder. He was convicted, but on appeal the court substituted a finding of manslaughter. He was sentenced to 8 years imprisonment.

There is no dispute in the public inquiry report as to the bare facts presented earlier. What is in dispute, and what forms the focus of the report, are essentially two issues: The first issue concerns the wisdom of the decision to return Maria to Mrs (and Mr) Kepple. The second concerns essentially the subsequent management of the case by the various agencies involved, but of course centrally by ESCC in carrying out the Supervision Order that was granted by Hove Juvenile Court in 1971.

The decision to return Maria

It is important to understand why East Sussex County Council took the decision that they did take in relation to Maria, that is, not to oppose the revocation of the Care Order. The minutes of a case discussion lasting over $1\frac{1}{2}$ hours made available to the subsequent Committee of Inquiry. The Inquiry Report sets out, in full, certain of the conclusions, which were that

It would seem whatever the decision was taken concerning Maria it would involve stress and trauma for her at some time. On balance it was felt that future plans should be directed towards her eventual return to her mother. It was recognised that while she remained with the Coopers she would continue to be the centre of conflict. It is unlikely that the Coopers will be able to deal well with her feelings in adolescence [*sic*], and it is possible that at that age she would herself decide to return to her mother. It should be easier for her to build relationships with the Kepple family and to take her place within [it] at a younger age, particularly considering the good emotional grounding she has received from the Coopers.

> (p. 19, paragraph 36, words bracketed are
> bracketed by the authors of the Report)

What the agency had in mind as 'an ideal solution' was for visits to the Kepples to be gradually increased. A 'gradual transfer from one family to another was envisaged' (p. 19, paragraph 36). This, however, was not possible in this case because of the animosity between the two families. Hence what they attempted was a

> Gradual changeover up to the point when the stress for Maria appeared to be becoming too great, i.e. contact with the Kepple family should be encouraged and increased to give Maria the opportunity of knowing them better before her sudden transfer to them. With this in view Mrs Kepple should be encouraged to delay her application for revocation and to go along with such a plan. If she insists on making such an application she should be opposed at this stage, but the long-term plan of Maria's return should be followed.
>
> (p. 19, paragraph 36)

The minutes of the case discussion conclude that, whatever action might be taken in the situation, either the Coopers or the Kepples would be hurt, but Maria's interests must be considered as a matter of 'paramount importance'.

The inquiry report acknowledges that in considering the case the social workers 'did not consider themselves in a position to make an unfettered decision' (p. 22, paragraph 42). This was because

> They operated within a legal and social system in which when a child was taken into care the expectation was not that she would remain in care until the age of eighteen but that she would return to her own family when the circumstances had improved. It was put to us ... that there was a strong presumption that the magistrates would return a child to the patent once the parent's fitness was proved, unless it could be clearly shown not to be in the best interests of the child.
>
> (p. 22, paragraph 42)

In other words the agency took the view that the magistrates would favour the claim of a biological parent over that of a foster parent, in the absence of strong evidence that they should not do so. The agency felt that they did not have such evidence. Hence if Mrs Kepple persisted with her application for revocation of the Care Order in relation to Maria, the agency genuinely believed she would be successful in so doing, because it would be argued by her solicitor that her living conditions had improved, that she was now in a stable relationship, and could seemingly cope with the children currently living with her (see p. 22). Mrs Kepple was quite entitled to make such and application *at any time* and was threatening to do so *at that time*. If she did so then the transfer would be immediate. Hence the agency were seeking to attempt to 'control the timing of such a move' (p. 22). The report points out that 'this view of the inevitability of Maria's return to her mother underlay much of the thinking in 1971 and profoundly affected the decisions taken and the management of the case' (p. 22, paragraph 42).

None of the above is in dispute in the Report of the Committee of Inquiry. However, what is a matter for comment and criticism within the Report is the wisdom of the decision not to oppose the revocation of the Care Order.

Both in the section of the Report entitled 'Narrative' and again in the conclusion of the majority report this decision is criticised. However, in the *minority report* by Ms Olive Stevenson the *decision is not criticised*. Hence, below, the criticisms made in the majority report are outlined first and then Ms Stevenson's objections to those criticisms are outlined.

Criticism of the decision to return Maria (majority report)

Paragraph 38 of the Report acknowledges that 'the most careful consideration was given to the situation as they saw it' (p. 20). However, in the same paragraph it is stated that there are two specific matters that were 'absolutely basic to any correct decision as to Maria's future'. They were thought to concern

> The question of whether it was really in Maria's best interests to be returned to her mother at all and ... the question of the true cause and depth of the trauma in Maria which it was envisaged would inevitably occur.

> (p. 20, paragraph 38)

The Report then suggests that the social workers were 'precluded' from making a correct decision right up until the juvenile court hearing. This was because they lacked information about *Mr Kepple*. In the words of the Report

> The social workers placed great stress upon the stable relationship between the Kepples. But the plain fact is that, apart from what Miss Lees was told by the Kepples themselves, neither of whom were truthful or reliable persons, nothing was known of Mr Kepple. His history, his family background, his record of employment, his pay packet, his habits, his character, his temperament, his philosophy of life, all were unknown save for what it was possible to observe of him and what Miss Lees was told by the Kepples.
>
> (p. 20, paragraph 39)

The Committee refers to the 'stringent requirements' that prospective foster parents were then required to satisfy under the appropriate regulations, and asks why Mr Kepple was not subjected to such scrutiny; and while it acknowledges that there was no statutory obligation to carry out such an investigation, the Committee nevertheless reports that 'commonsense would dictate at least some similar investigation. It is no answer in this case to point out the difficulties involved because the attempt was never made. If Maria's interests were paramount, it should have been' (p. 21, paragraph 39). The Committee also refers to Mr Kepple's previous four convictions involving (minor) violence, none of which involved children and all of which were 'a long time previously'.

In paragraph 45 the Committee members set down the parameters in terms of which they are prepared to criticise social workers. They acknowledge that they had been urged not to criticise social workers 'if they had made reasoned judgements, in accordance with contemporary standards of practice amongst their colleagues and the judgements were arrived at in the light of the available information' (p. 23), and therefore indicate that they will not do this.

However, they do feel able to criticise the crucial issue of Maria's return to her mother since they feel that even though a reasoned decision was precluded, 'a decision was taken nevertheless' (p. 23, paragraph 45). The implication here is that they can criticise the social workers even within the above remit since they took a decision which was not 'reasoned', because they were not able to take a 'reasoned' one. The further implication is, of course, that the situation should have been further and more fully investigated. The assumption appears to be that such further investigation would produce evidence for the final outcome which, with hindsight, was clear to all concerned.

In one particular aspect the Committee members also feel able to criticise 'contemporary standard practice itself' (p. 23, paragraph 45). This concerns the 'acceptance of an unduly high degree of trauma to a child in the process of being transplanted'.

The criticisms of the decision to return Maria, then, revolve around the following clearly defined issues. In the first place the social workers are criticised for simply setting too much store by the 'stable relationship' in which Mrs Kepple was at the time involved, even if they believed that a magistrates court would take a similar view. They were criticised for not establishing the true cause and depth of Maria's trauma, and the implication here is that her trauma concerned not confusion as to where her loyalties lay, as was suggested in Ms Lees' court report, but rather that Maria was all too clear about that, that is, she was happy with her 'Mum and Dad' (the Coopers) and unhappy and afraid at her mother's (Mrs Kepple). They are also criticised for sanctioning this level of trauma in any event, and also for not investigating the background of Mr Kepple, in terms of vetting him, in the way that any prospective foster parent would be vetted. The assumption that Maria would find it more difficult later, and therefore less difficult sooner, to rejoin her mother was also criticised. The implication here is that the assumption was groundless and that expert opinion, if consulted, would have told them so.

Ms Olive Stevenson's minority report

This report forms chapter 5 of the total Report. It is concerned only with the period covered earlier, that is, the period up until the revocation of the Care Order. In her letter to the then Secretary of State she has this to say:

> I differ very considerably from my colleagues in the interpretation of Maria's situation and the social workers' actions during those years. As a former social worker in childcare, I have had constantly in mind the possible impact of this report on relations between *natural and foster parents in this country, and thus on the children involved*. These relationships are often complicated and highly charged emotionally. In Maria's case, they were particularly so because of the network of relatives. In my view it can only do harm to children in care or under supervision, if these issues are over simplified; and this I believe my colleagues have done.
>
> (p. 7, paragraph 248, my emphasis)

Ms Stevenson in the introduction to her report proper argues that her colleagues have not done justice 'to the difficulties which Ms Lees and her colleagues inherited in 1969' (p. 88).

Ms Stevenson offers a more detailed narrative than do her colleagues concerning the period in question. She considers the period of Maria's early history as a part of that. She offers three reasons for doing so. In the first place she is concerned to present a 'fair picture', which cannot be done, in her view, 'without an account of the earlier history...which conveys the complexity' (p. 88, paragraph 248). Second, she wishes to demonstrate 'the care and attention given to Maria in this period', and third, she feels that only such a detailed account could enable her to consider the strengths as well as the weaknesses involved in the care and supervision of Maria. She points out that the brief of the inquiry was not simply to 'find fault' but to 'examine the care and supervision' of Maria (see p. 88, paragraph 248).

The discourse of maternal deprivation in the minority report

Ms Stevenson's analysis of the events, which attempts to give a fuller and more sympathetic account of the social worker's activities, is explicitly in parts located within the discourse of maternal deprivation. She uses this discourse in order to cast doubt on her colleagues' view in relation to their apparent assumption that Maria's trauma upon leaving the Coopers was simply and solely a result of her affection for them, and that Mrs Kepple's desire for her return was simply to use her as a drudge.

She achieves this by use of the following steps. In the first place (paragraph 249) she recalls that the first trauma in Maria's life might have been her initial separation from her mother when she was deposited with Mrs Cooper at the age of 5 months. She then presents two reasons for Mrs Kepple's removing Maria, and taking her to someone less suitable than the Coopers, when Maria was 14 months old. She suggests that Mrs Kepple may have obtained a 'particular gratification' in caring for infants, and this may have explained her many pregnancies – she had placed Maria with the Coopers in the first place because she was stressed and overwrought as a result of her bereavement in relation to Mr Colwell. On this analysis, part of her desire ultimately to have Maria back was 'a deep regret, even anger at having missed a part of Maria's infancy which would have given her much satisfaction. It may be that in 1972 she was *unconsciously* envisaging the return of her *baby*'

(p. 89, paragraph 249, my emphasis). Her removal of Maria at the age of 14 months was perhaps because of her 'growing resentment of Maria's attachment to Mr and Mrs Cooper' (p. 89, paragraph 250). Nevertheless, her removal from a mother figure, that is, Mrs Cooper, at the age of 14 months is a further trauma because 'there is overwhelming evidence from the literature that a sudden separation from a "mother figure"... may have profound repercussions on a child's emotional state' (p. 89, paragraph 251). However, over the page, the 'may' in the earlier paragraph becomes a 'must'. It is suggested that 'this *must* have been a profoundly disturbing experience' (p. 90, paragraph 251).

The conclusion from the above is delivered in the next paragraph when she states that 'the possible relevance of this experience to Maria's subsequent behaviour, when separated from Mrs Cooper, cannot be overlooked' (p. 90, paragraph 252).

Hence by use of the discourse of maternal deprivation, Ms Stevenson casts potential doubt in relation to her colleagues' interpretation of Maria's behaviour in running away from Mrs Kepple's and returning to relatives of the Coopers. Maria had had a number of separations, they were traumatic, here was another one and she voted with her feet. This compares with the implied view of her colleagues, which was that, while the reason for her behaviour was not fully investigated, and it should have been, the idea that there was a simple confusion of loyalties on Maria's behalf, which was held by the social worker in her court report, was based on insufficient evidence, and an equally good or even better interpretation was that Maria was devoted to the Coopers and afraid and upset at living with Mrs (and, of course, Mr) Kepple. The distinction here is a fine one. Ms Stevenson is implying that given her early history Maria would react badly to *any* separation.

She also questions the decision to return Maria immediately to the Coopers, under the Place of Safety Order, after Mrs Kepple had deposited Maria with an unsuitable person at age 14 months. While on the face of it the decision was obvious, she makes the point that Mrs Kepple had expressed a preference for a residential nursery. Avoiding further 'maternal deprivation' through the use of such a resource was in the social worker's mind at the time, as was Maria's good relationship with the Coopers. Ms Stevenson appreciates all of this. However, for all of that she wonders if

> Viewed in retrospect, it is possible to argue that in this humane and seemingly obvious choice lay the seeds of the tragic 'tug of *love*' which was to follow. Mrs Kepple, in removing Maria, had given an

indication of the way the wind would blow and it is worth noting that at the point when the choice was made she herself expressed a preference for residential care.

(p. 91, paragraph 255, my emphasis)

The family feud

Olive Stevenson then outlines in detail the fact of the 'feud' between various factions of the 'family network'. The evidence of relatives, she says, led her to believe that the 'network of family communications and interactions on both sides was exceedingly complex' (see p. 91, paragraph 256). There were apparently numerous phone calls concerning difficulties of access on both sides – sometimes Mrs Kepple did not collect Maria on time, and at other times she did, only to find her out. Mrs Kepple also, for instance, refused to consent to the christening arranged by the Coopers, 'ostensibly on religious grounds' (p. 93, paragraph 263). There was concern that the Coopers' relationship to Maria was 'over intense' (see p. 93, paragraph 266). The origins of the feud appeared to pre-date the fostering of Maria by the Coopers, and extend across generations.

From all of the factors outlined earlier, Ms Stevenson concluded that

Although varying in intensity, Mrs Kepple's interest in Maria and resentment of her placement with Mr and Mrs Cooper was ever present from 1966 onwards.

Secondly, Mrs Cooper was always disturbed and upset by Mrs Kepple's interventions.

Thirdly, the wider families on both sides played a significant part in the difficulties.

Fourthly, the social workers were perceptive of the feelings of Maria, Mrs Cooper and Mrs Kepple and were struggling to find ways of achieving rapprochement for Maria's sake.

(p. 97, paragraph 275)

She immediately adds that this attempt to achieve rapprochement was not with any 'specific intention of returning Maria to her mother', but that they believed it to be important 'for her emotional welfare'. She wonders, however, with 'hindsight', whether they were 'over optimistic' in thinking that these 'deep seated difficulties would be amenable to help'. She also adds that 'perhaps they had to believe that', given their decision to leave Maria with Mrs Cooper in 1966 (p. 97, paragraph 275).

Paragraphs 276–94 cover the narrative up until the point in the case discussion in which the social workers decide not to oppose the revocation of the Care Order. They centrally concern the way in which Maria was at the centre of, and in some senses like a pawn in, an extended family feud, and the efforts made by Ms Lees (the social worker) to understand the feelings of all concerned and to attempt to mediate. They also concern the period when it firmly emerged that Mrs Kepple was intending to legally seek the return of her daughter, and the efforts that were made to slow down the timing of this event and to speed up contact between Maria and her mother in order that Maria might get to know her better.

Paragraph 294 concerns the social worker's 'understandable worry about the situation. It was suggested to her by her senior that she write down all the negatives in the situation. Her conclusion in this note-like list is that 'given personalities and relationships... no happy solution possible. Maria... [was] bound to suffer' (p. 103).

In the following paragraph Ms Stevenson reports that Ms Lees records 'somewhat despairingly' that 'casework help seems ineffective and my role is more that of a mediator between all parties' (p. 104).

Paragraph 296 (p. 104) sees Maria refusing to visit her mother for the second time that month, and Mr Cooper carrying Maria to the car, while being bitten and scratched by her. Ms Lees concludes that there is 'absolutely no question' of persevering with the planned visit.

Maria was placed at 'home on trial' on 22 October 1971 and she again ran away from her mother's house to relatives and demanded of Ms Lees that she be taken back to the Coopers. Ms Lees thought that she 'calmed down' upon 'the appearance of her mother' (p. 107, paragraph 306).

On 17 November of that same year the juvenile court revoked the Care Order. Ms Stevenson is not critical of Ms Lees' report to the magistrates, feeling that, though she did not mention all the running away episodes, nevertheless the situation was clearly outlined to the court. The magistrates did not seek evidence from Mr Kepple and they, unlike the social workers, are not criticised for this in the majority report. Ms Stevenson points out the formal nature of court reports, and the requirements of evidence which do not permit of speculation. She also reminds a reader that it is custom and practice for parents to see such reports and that 'these factors make them properly cautious' (p. 107, paragraph 309). She adds that nevertheless it might have been 'wise for Ms Lees to air more fully some of her reservations about Mr Kepple that she had expressed in her case notes' unless these doubts had by that time been resolved (p. 107, paragraph 309).

From all of the earlier, Ms Stevenson concludes that the case was extraordinarily complex and, of course, rapidly changing, and that, given those factors, the social worker's records display a 'better than average quality in their perceptiveness of the feelings of all concerned in this agonising situation and in their patient attempts to improve relations' (p. 108, paragraph 312).

In relation to the decision not to oppose Maria's return to live with her mother and stepfather, which of course was a central area in which the social workers were criticised by Ms Stevenson's colleagues, she makes several points. In the first place she reminds a reader that her colleagues accepted that the social workers were operating within a social and legal framework, and that a strong presumption that the magistrates would themselves return Maria was not in itself unreasonable given the fact that 'until very recently the courts have sought to balance the welfare of the child with the rights of natural parents and it has not always been clear that the former is paramount' (p. 109, paragraph 314).

The 'blood tie'

Ms Stevenson also comments on the issue of the 'blood tie', over which she feels there is 'much confusion' (p. 109, paragraph 315). She argues that social workers do not generally accept that an emotional relationship, taking precedence over other emotional relationships, inevitably exists between a child and a biological parent merely because of consanguinity. The issue is, in her view, much more related to the question of any given child's identity and good self-image. There are, in her view, two elements involved in this. In the first place a child should know who her/his parents are and, second, her/his view of them should not be adversely coloured by adults who may be parenting the child, since the children may then have a poor image of themselves because of the belief that they come from 'bad stock' (p. 109, paragraph 315).

In relation to Maria's 'true feelings' and the interpretation that the social workers gave to her behaviour, Ms Stevenson points out that Maria's feelings 'fluctuated wildly', and she adds that it was inevitable that 'she would be affected by the attitudes and behaviour of those with her at any time', especially when they were competing 'for her affection, sometimes in a not very controlled or sensitive way' (p. 110, paragraph 317). The social workers were faced with allegation and counter-allegation from people known to be feuding over Maria and wider long-standing matters, and also with Maria's seemingly inconsistent behaviour. Ms Stevenson feels that it was therefore unfair to criticise

Ms Lees and her agency, in retrospect, for not making a different interpretation to the one which they did make. She does however feel that the 'running away episodes' should have been probed 'more deeply', and points out that they are less fully recorded than some of the visits. She adds that 'such behaviour is very unusual in young children and I am not satisfied that Ms Lees took them sufficiently seriously' (p. 111, paragraph 317).

Social work as an independent discipline

The minority report also dissents from the view, expressed in the majority report, that Ms Lees should have made a psychiatric referral, since to insist that she did so would be tantamount to denying her 'a basic tool of her own trade' (p. 111, paragraph 318). She also points out that a referral was not made at the point at which her colleagues thought it should be, simply because the agency considered Maria's reactions to be normal and not pathological. They did not rule out potential psychiatric help at any later stage, only at that particular stage.

Olive Stevenson does not dissent from the majority report in relation to the enquiries which should be made of potential stepfathers, while noting the difficulties involved in making enquiries of the police, etc. She points out that Ms Lees' conduct was in line with standard social-work practice, a standard practice, though, 'which could be improved'. She also points out that Mr Kepple's minor convictions, acquired many years before his involvement with Mrs Kepple and subsequently Maria, 'could be matched by many other parents'. Hence she feels that even if this had been uncovered it need not have affected the decision to return Maria to her mother, and in fact probably would not have done so (p. 113, paragraph 232). However, in paragraph 331, she suggests that 'there would have been much to be gained if Maria had had a considerably longer period home on trial' prior to the revocation of the court order. This would have focused the social worker into a closer consideration of the situation if there was to be a further hearing to assess that period prior to the revocation of the order. She adds, however, that she accepts that social workers under stress, 'as Miss Lees was at that time', are 'bound to be affected in their priorities, by certain external demands, such as court reports' (p. 115, paragraph 331).

The conclusions of the minority report

Ms Stevenson has three paragraphs headed 'Conclusions', and in them she states that she shares her colleagues' views on the 'failure of various systems for which we all must take share of responsibility'. She feels that the most 'serious failures in this sad story were in communications within and between agencies'. She was 'perturbed' that some who gave evidence to the enquiry had an 'implicit assumption that the responsibility for efficient communication lay solely with the social workers rather than with all the official persons concerned with Maria's welfare' (p. 115, paragraph 332).

She is in agreement in relation to the events subsequent to Maria's return to her mother, but not in relation to events before it. She points out the stress and overload that East Sussex social workers were facing in that period, and, while she says that 'there is no excuse in professional terms to fail to supervise adequately', nevertheless she adds that

> A society which is compassionate to Maria, to Mr and Mrs Cooper and, hopefully, also to Mr and Mrs Kepple, should extend similar sympathy to those whom it employs to perform tasks of the utmost difficulty and complexity, under conditions of great strain.
>
> (p. 115, paragraph 332)

She concludes by saying that she does not think that a 'hierarchy of censure is appropriate'. She adds that there was 'much that was excellent' in the work of East Sussex Social Services Department, and that 'all played a part in the tragedy, including the schools' (p. 115, paragraph 334).

Familialism and the 'tug of love'

Quite clearly at the centre of the Maria Colwell case is the issue of familialism, and within that the issue of the claims of the biological against the social/psychological parent. The social workers took the decision that they did in relation to the non-opposition to the revocation of a Care Order, because while they themselves may not have agreed, they genuinely thought that within given parameters – that is, providing it could not be illustrated in court that there was good reason *not* to do so – then the magistrates court would entrust the care of a child to a biological parent over a foster parent, even if the child seemed happy enough to live with the foster parent.

It is not only that 'all things being equal' this was what they thought a court would do, since all things were manifestly *not* equal in this case. If they thought that all things *were* equal they would not have requested a Supervision Order in relation to Maria upon her joining the household of Mrs Kepple. The social workers themselves, as their case notes cited both in the majority and minority report illustrate, were worried. Nevertheless they took the view that their worries alone would not sufficiently impress the court, and they were not in possession of what they considered to be adequate evidence. Hence in the light of the above it appeared that they thought that a biological parent's rights would be upheld even if there was a very differential track record in relation to the care of the child. This was based on experience at the time.

The issue of familialism itself is important since the question of residential care was ruled out. Of course there were reasons for this: for example the good relationship that existed between Maria and the Coopers. However, it is also true, as the minority report illustrates, that such a move may have removed Maria from the centre of a competition for her affection and ultimately for her physical presence in one particular household and not another. The move to residential care was ruled out also on the grounds of avoiding (further) maternal deprivation. This discourse still had, and sometimes still has, a very strong hold within social work. This is further illustrated by Ms Stevenson's no doubt at times politically skilful use of the discourse, in breaking down the obviousness implied in the majority report's interpretation of Maria's resistance to separation from Mrs and Mr Cooper.

What is important about this is that there was an obviousness about the fact that a child should live in a 'family'. The only question was: which one? Indeed in order to have a hope of regaining the care of Maria (and quite independently of whether this was wise or not), Mrs Kepple had to present herself as a new family. Mrs Kepple had a new house, and a new man, and she had held onto both of them for long enough to be thought of as a 'stable family unit'. Before that time Mrs Kepple would have had *no chance* of regaining her child, and yet after it she had, as far as the social workers involved could see, *every chance*, even if they themselves didn't like that fact.

Mr Kepple and the court

The court saw no reason to cross-examine Mr Kepple, notwithstanding the fact that the social worker did in fact discuss his relationship to Maria and her return to Mrs Kepple with him, and she was concerned at his apparent bewilderment that this could be a matter for discussion at all.

Now whether or not it would have been wise for Ms Lees to share these concerns with the magistrate's court, and whether or not she should have gone into this at a greater depth, it is nevertheless important to remember that the court itself apparently saw no reason why this should be done. It should also be remembered that there was no statutory obligation on either the court or the social worker to do so. It is hard therefore to escape the conclusion that the business of child rearing was seen as overwhelmingly in the main the task of a woman, and that her task included the nurturing and the protection of her child.

The social workers and their agency were criticised for not asking questions that the court seemingly saw no reason themselves to ask, and which neither had any statutory obligation to ask. All this is, of course, firmly within the parameters of the historic discourse of child protection: 'the Family' and a woman's role within it are taken as given.

However, the familial ideology impacting on the discourse misses a crucial point, that is, it is a man who killed Maria. Faced with tragic consequences, in the life (and death) of a real person the Law must ask: 'what has gone wrong, who is responsible, what must change?' The bearers of the discourse are not conscious of the contradiction to their ideology and discourse that these events provided, though they speak for and on behalf of the Law. In other words the bearers of the discourse cannot say that the discourse is itself at fault, since they see their discourse and the unconscious familial ideology brought to it as the truth. Nevertheless as a result of such an inquiry the discourse may, and often will, paradoxically, be shielded by the production of a discursive shift, which in turn contributes to a change in the law. It does so in this case by making the interests of the child central.

In relation to the general duty of local authorities when making decisions relating to children in their care, the 1975 Children Act amended the 1948 Children Act. Under the 1948 Act the duty was to further the best interests of any child in their care and to 'afford him the opportunity for the proper development of his character and abilities' (see Terry 1979: 85). The 1975 Act insists that

> In reaching any decision relating to a child in their care, a local authority shall give *first consideration* to the need to safeguard and promote the welfare of the child throughout his childhood; and shall so far as is practicable ascertain the wishes and feelings of the child regarding the decision and give due consideration to them, having regard to his age and understanding.
>
> (Section 59, quoted in Terry
> 1979: 85)

Also, in disputes concerning the biological parent as against a foster parent, the interests of the child are said to be paramount. Perhaps this is as it should be. But the important point is that it was not always thus. This can be illustrated by again quoting Terry (1979) who; in her book *A Guide to the Children Act 1975*, points out that

> Part 11 of the 1975 Act also contains amendments to the Children and Young Persons Act 1969. One of the most significant of these amendments is the introduction of separate representation for a child in court where there is a conflict of interests between a child and his parents in certain proceedings under the Act.
>
> (p. 97)

She later adds that

> The Maria Colwell case must spring to everyone's mind as an example of where there was a conflict of interests and an independent spokesman representing the child's circumstances and feelings to the court might have prevented the discharge of the care order, and thereby avoided the ensuing tragedy.
>
> (p. 98)

This is important, because without an understanding of the way in which this legal change took place, one might, especially if one only had as a guide an analysis which gave a moral panic the central role in increasing concern for the rights of the child, have at best only a partial analysis. This of course would be particularly so if a category mistake was involved in linking child abuse to an existing panic about something quite different. Such an analysis leads a person away from grasping the necessity to consider carefully the discourse which is already present in existing legislation. When fault lines appear in the existing legislation, that same discourse may be further emphasised and often further enshrined in new legislation.

Jennifer Terry (1979) *in her use of language is* again revealing in this context. Of the power vested in the Secretary of State to institute a statutory inquiry she writes that

> The Maria Colwell case drew attention to the fact that the Secretary of State for Social Services had no statutory power to cause an inquiry to be held, and therefore had no power to subpoena witnesses, require the production of documents or take evidence on oath. The Act *puts this right* by section 96.
>
> (p. 119, my emphasis)

In other words the Act has 'put right' that which is wrong. The Law, and the people chosen to investigate what has gone wrong with it, do not, as such, panic. Newspapers may do so, people at a general level may do so, individual policemen might and do panic – as might and do their superior officers. Social workers may panic and no doubt many do, and their agency managers may well make panicky decisions in relation to childcare issues, especially when they have seen their colleagues publicly criticised for appearing to be chary in intervening into a situation. But the process of making legislation is far more calm and methodical than this. It methodically attempts to 'put right' that which it finds wrong – even if what is wrong is an aspect of its own discourse. This understanding induces one to pay attention to the specificity of such discourse. This does not mean of course that those who sit on committees of inquiry, etc. do not read newspapers; no doubt they do, and no doubt some of them are influenced by them. Nevertheless, and this is the important point, the newspaper editors write newspaper editorials – they do not, moral panics notwithstanding, write the Law. This is a far more incremental process.

Chapter 8

Back to the future

This chapter summarises and restates the analysis contained in the previous chapters of this book, and it also offers some conclusions from this analysis. The conclusions to be drawn from the book fall into two areas. In the first place there is what can be concluded from the detailed analysis of the various documents considered. Second, there are further conclusions, albeit more tentative ones, to be drawn concerning the issue of discourse analysis, on the one hand, and the concept of ideology on the other. These will be dealt with under separate headings.

CONCLUSIONS FROM THE ANALYSIS OF THE VARIOUS DOCUMENTS CONSIDERED

From the earliest days of social work, indeed since the COS (see Jones 1983, cited in Chapter 1 of this book), there has been a discourse of prevention. In the case of the COS, it was pauperism that was to be prevented by the application of 'scientific' knowledge. This depoliticised the issue of pauperism and poverty by targeting specific 'scientific' interventions at particular sections of the working class, and not poverty itself. By the mid-1920s (see Chapter 5 of this book), cruelty, neglect and delinquency became the issue for prevention. There has been a discourse of technical intervention in the name of prevention since the foundation of the social-work profession. The discourse of treatment against punishment which emanated in the main from the Home Office Children's Department and which was responsible, by means of its own influence upon any particular government of the day, in constructing childcare law, called forth the social-work profession that we know today. In so doing it produced, right at the centre of that activity, a number of contradictions, tensions and even 'impossibilities'.

For instance, the discourse called for the prevention of juvenile delinquency, and suggested that poverty was at the root of it, and then immediately ignored the question of poverty. It focused instead upon 'the' family, and interventions within it. Such interventions were either into the subjectivity of delinquent working-class children, or their parents, or both. The discourse at best produced only a partial response and therefore only a partial solution: and partial solutions, far from solving problems, often make them worse. This is all the more true if it is not noticed, recognised or acknowledged that the proffered solution is partial and also if it nevertheless makes great claims for itself: for example, the prevention of juvenile delinquency and, as a result of that, the reduction of adult crime (see Chapter 6).

The ideological element in the discourse of familialism

For this discourse, the family is both the problem and the solution. Trouble occurs in 'problem families' and 'families with problems'. On the other hand, 'the' family itself appears to be above criticism. There are a number of negative consequences of this very sharp familial focus. For instance it constructs a notion of a singular family, essentially the heterosexual, white European nuclear family. Other family or household forms therefore become invisible, or problematised. Thus it is an ethnocentric, unconsciously ideological notion of the family, which is brought to the text of the discourse, and which is therefore unconscious of differing cultural traditions of rearing children. In radically dichotomising the 'problem family' and the 'family with a problem' from all other families, the discourse minimalises the problems and indeed the potential oppression of women and children in the families which are not seen as either 'problem families' or 'families with a problem'. The notion of a singular family is simplistic and flawed. Hence the solution which the discourse offers can only be partial. Furthermore the 'social science' knowledge mobilised is simply insufficiently 'hard/sound' to be able to predict and prevent the problems that it is supposed to predict and prevent.

In other words what was offered was a promise, which in itself, even with the best knowledge and the best technology of intervention, and the most highly trained personnel, would remain a very tall order indeed. This was greatly compounded by the partial nature of the analysis of the problem. All of this was again further compounded by the idealisation of a singular, white, heterosexual nuclear family and by the resulting reductionist understanding of delinquency and neglect as stemming everywhere from problems within the family.

The placing upon local authorities of the duty to prevent care proceedings, and to investigate where there is suspicion of the need for such proceedings, all within the above discursively and ideologically constructed contradictions, inevitably produces tragic failures. Indeed it is a matter for surprise that, relatively speaking, it produces so few of them. When such tragic failures give rise to 'moral panic', as they no doubt do, the panic reaction often only serves to further obscure the discursively and ideologically constructed boundaries of the issue. This in itself may lead to giving a particular 'moral panic' too great a determining influence in the production of future legislation (see Chapter 7).

Ideology and discourse

A more nuanced account of these particular historical moments may be assisted by a consideration of the question of ideology and discourse in relation to the above. What is required is a version of both discourse analysis and ideology which can fruitfully operate together in a non-reductionist way. Fairclough (1989) (see Chapter 2 of this book) offers such a version of discourse analysis, which mobilises the work of Antonio Gramsci. He suggests that

> Ideology is most effective when its workings are least visible. If one becomes aware that a particular aspect of common sense is sustaining power relations at one's own expense, it ceases to be common sense, and may cease to have the capacity to sustain power inequalities, i.e. to function ideologically. And invisibility is achieved when ideologies are brought to discourse not as explicit elements of the text, but as the background assumptions which on the one hand lead the text producer to 'textualise' the world in a particular way, and on the other hand lead the interpreter to interpret the text in a particular way. Texts do not typically spout ideology. They so position the interpreter through their cues that she brings ideologies to the interpretation of texts – and reproduces them in the process.
>
> (p. 85)

This can be seen in the discourse of treatment against punishment contained in the various Reports of the Home Office Children's Committee, and also in the development of that same discourse as emanating from the Curtis Committee, which is considered in Chapter 5 of this book.

For instance, via an examination of aspects of the discourse of the Home Office Children's Department, it can be illustrated that, by 1938, there was already a very high level of over-promising taking place, and this had serious implications in that it ultimately constructed social work as, in an almost literal sense, an 'impossible' profession – at least as an extremely tall order. The discourse of treatment, as opposed to punishment, acknowledges poverty as causal in terms of delinquency. However, it does not permit this explanation of the problem to become any part of the solution to the problem. Instead the focus is once again shifted to individual interventions into the subjectivities of young working-class people: training, treatment, rehabilitation and ultimately prediction and prevention.

The problem, of course, is simply that if it really is the case that, as the 1923 Home Office Children's Report (HMSO 1923) suggests, 'poverty seems to be undoubtedly at the bottom of much of the delinquency among children' (p. 5) or, in the words of the 1938 Children's Branch Report (HMSO 1938), that

> It would be more correct to attribute their downfall to the unsatisfactory social conditions which unfortunately still exist in London and in our great industrial areas, for it is from these that the children of the approved school are mainly gathered.
>
> (p. 43)

then it must also be true that in order to fulfil this big promise of reducing the level of adult crime, the question of the causes of poverty and unsatisfactory social conditions must necessarily be addressed. Yet the discourse nowhere does this. In moving, as the discourse does, from any recognition or response to poverty, to an individualised intervention, it depoliticises the issue of both deprivation and delinquency. This depoliticisation, that is, the shift from the social system to individual technical intervention, produces a promise which cannot be fulfilled outside a re-politicisation of the issue, and even this in itself would be no guarantee.

As is suggested above, it is not the case that the discourse 'spouts ideology'. The shift from the social system to a technology of individual intervention is accomplished by a forgetting. It is a forgetting that a reader of the text, like the author of the text, would not notice if 'common sense' had relegated the absence of that which was forgotten to the status of something about which nothing could be done. The forgetting of poverty seems to work like this in the texts under consideration. It is clearly acknowledged as causal but then, without explanation, excuse or apology, it disappears as quickly as it arrives. This central absence, just like the emperor's new clothes, is not apparent to the emperor, the absence is not missed and it is not seen as absence until someone dares to point it out.

In other words, the ideology is implicit. It depends, just like the emperor's new clothes, on a shared assumption. The common-sense ideology of the text has to meet the common-sense ideology of the reader. If it does not, then the absence is plain and the game is up. Similarly with the extreme familialism of the Curtis Committee, it is seen simply as obvious, natural, mere common sense; it requires no explanation.

Of course, there are many explanations for forgetfulness, even ideological forgetfulness. It is not the case that the only cause of ideological forgetting is that it makes no (common) sense to remember what it is that is forgotten, because nothing can be done about it, or because it is fair, or because it is natural or otherwise inevitable etc. Eagleton (1991) (see Chapter 2 of this book) points out that

> Freud has little to say directly of ideology; but it is very probable that what he points to as the fundamental mechanisms of the physical life are the structural devices of ideology as well. Projection, displacement, sublimation, condensation, repression, idealisation, substitution, rationalisation, disavowal; all these are at work in the text of ideology, as much as in dream and fantasy; and this is one of the richest legacies Freud has bequeathed to the critique of ideological consciousness.
>
> (p. 185)

It is, of course, also perfectly possible that all of this is a conscious and fully rational affair in which, in the case in question, the originator of the discourse in question, while feeling that poverty ought at least to be acknowledged, nevertheless feels it imprudent to dwell on that which would inconvenience or otherwise displease the political masters for whom it was produced. In which case we would be dealing with a case of suppression and not repression; after all, the originator or bearer of a discourse does not have to be the self-deluded dupe of his own discourse, and may well not be. For instance, Mr A. H. Norris, who was at the head of the Children's Branch of the Home Office through a 21-year period, and 'served' therefore a Conservative government, a Liberal government, a National government, and a Labour government, was no doubt skilled in the matter of avoiding offending the political sensibilities of his 'masters', to whom he was ever the 'obedient servant' while nevertheless pursuing, give or take some shifts in emphasis and the occasional linguistic transformation, his own, or his department's own agenda.

Ideology may of course be at work in disrupting the text in other ways too. What is clear is that there is a 'performance contradiction' in the discourse. In other words there is a difference between what is said and what is then done. Some aspects of this contradiction can be explained by a recognition that

> What makes a dominant ideology powerful – its ability to intervene in the consciousness of those it subjects, appropriating and rein-flecting their experience – is also what tends to make it internally heterogeneous and consistent. A successful ruling ideology, as we have seen, must engage significantly with genuine wants, needs and desires; but this is also its Achilles heel, forcing it to recognise an 'other' to itself and inscribing this otherness as a potentially disruptive force within its own forms.
>
> (Eagleton 1991: 45)

In the discourse under consideration the genuine need is an economic one – it is poverty, and it is the 'other' of the discourse, and its Achilles heel. It therefore renders the discourse internally inconsistent, but it also nevertheless makes the discourse more powerful, precisely because it appears to acknowledge and recognise poverty. Hence the perform-ance contradiction may be explained in this way: that is, poverty is consciously acknowledged, which legitimises the discourse, making it visibly 'liberal', but it is also simultaneously suppressed, leaving the field open for theories of treatment and not punishment, which is the real conscious business of the discourse; however, this leaves the discourse internally inconsistent.

IN SUMMARY

What appears to be overlooked in much of the existing academic literature, and by policy makers, in the field of British childcare legisla-tion, up to and including the 2004 Children Act, is the ever-present tension between two discourses. These discourses, which are on the one hand the discourse of punishment and on the other the discourse of treat-ment, are apparent from the beginning of twentieth-century childcare legislation in Britain. The discourse of treatment ultimately translates into a statutory duty laid upon social workers for the prevention of child abuse in all of its forms. At the same time the duty to detect and intervene in abusive situations, sometimes by removing children from abusive parents, remains. This leaves social workers treading a 'discursively constructed tightrope' which can have tragic consequences in which too much emphasis is placed on one pole of this dichotomy at the expense of the other. This leads them to be exposed to the charge of either too little or too much intervention and thus places them, at least at times, in a near impossible situation.

The discourse of prevention leads to an emphasis upon familialism: that is, an underlying assumption that, apart from sad exceptions, children are always and everywhere best looked after in families, and all other alternatives are seen as a last resort. Where there are tragedies as a result of the above, the Public Inquiries which often result, and the subsequent legislative changes that they in turn often bring in their wake, do not recognise this discursively constructed dilemma. The result of this is that the dilemma is often compounded by further legislation. Via discursive shifts, new legislation may emphasise one of the two discourses. An example would be that the 1989 Children Act emphasises working in partnership with parents and families; however, whatever the particular emphasis between these two discourses, the legislation never entirely abandon either one of them. Hence, albeit with a shift in emphasis, the 'discursively constructed tightrope' always remains.

This sadly remains the case in relation to the 2004 Children Act (see Chapter 3 of this book). This is because Lord Laming's Inquiry Report into the tragic death of Victoria Climbié sees the 1989 Children Act as essentially sound legislation and leaves the wider contradictions within social work un-analysed, thus leaving the competing discourses, and the resultant conflicting duties of social workers, intact. Lord Laming focuses instead on the issue of the better implementation of the 1989 Children Act.

BACK TO THE FUTURE

In the context of the 'here and now' it is important to consider and outline the implications of the work of this book for social-work practice in the light of the 2004 Children Act, and the 1989 Children Act (see Chapters 3 and 4). The central role of social workers in terms of statutory responsibility for prevention, rehabilitation and detection, outlined in the 1989 Children Act, remains essentially undisturbed by the legislation of 2004. The focus of that legislation, following the Laming Report, is on the better managerial implementation of the 1989 Act. Hence, the critical consideration of the 1989 Children Act, which is the subject of Chapter 4, remains relevant.

As discussed throughout, this book has suggested that it is the tension between a legislative duty to intervene into 'the family' where there is believed to be a risk of (in the case of the 1989 Act) 'significant harm' to the child, and also the duty to promote 'the family' as the best place to look after children, which necessarily involves the prediction and prevention of child abuse and which leads periodically, episodically, but nevertheless inevitably, to the kind of opposing outcomes involved in both the Maria Colwell case and the Cleveland case and other subsequent cases like them.

In other words it is not too little or too much intervention which is the major issue, it is rather the imperative legislative duty, of specifically the social services departments and their successors, to intervene for often very differing and conflicting reasons which leads inevitably at times to, quite simply, the wrong intervention at the wrong time.

Furthermore, the conflicting demands and their discursive roots within nearly a century of British childcare legislation rarely, if ever, become visible at all. Hence this is not recognised as a problem, and individual social workers and their agencies and managers are therefore themselves held largely responsible for these negative consequences. In this sense, the Children Act 2004 can be seen, in an important sense, as more of the same. Of course none of this means that child abuse is not in itself requiring of serious attention. What is, however, under consideration are the discourses within the legislation that form and condition such intervention.

'Authoritarian familialism?'

While broadly part of the same general ideological trajectory as noted above, the kind of familialism involved in the 1989 Act is clearly also different from the essentially social democratic familialism which reached a high-water mark in the 1969 Children and Young Persons Act, in which great faith was placed in preventative and curative expertise, however misplaced that faith ultimately appeared to be (see Chapter 5 of this book). The brand of familialism involved in the 1989 Act has a more authoritarian ring; it is a question of a responsibility and not of a right. Hence the Act uses the term 'parental responsibility'. A responsibility is something that one is obliged to fulfil. It is not the case that parents, or for that matter children, are seen as having rights which the State will assist them in maintaining via services and material assistance for parents, caretakers and children.

On the contrary, it is a situation in which parents have responsibilities and the State will offer monetary resources only in rare circumstances, and it will intervene (in partnership with parents) only where there is a risk of significant harm. Perhaps, therefore, this could be termed 'authoritarian familialism' in order to differentiate it from the 'social democratic' familialism of earlier legislation. The seemingly genderless nature of parents which occurs throughout the discourse also obscures the fact that the burden of responsibility for caring for a family falls overwhelmingly upon women as mothers and also obscures the fact that, overwhelmingly, physical and sexual abuse is perpetrated by men upon girls.

Of course the question is not simply a question of a simple competition between 'pro-family' and 'anti-family' discourse. There are different approaches to this question and indeed a 'pro-family' social democratic focus would involve, at the minimum, significantly enhanced material support for working-class families. Hence it is important to recognise that the 'pro-family' focus of the 1989 Children Act is specific. It imposes specific responsibilities while, the concept of 'partnership' notwithstanding, offering little or nothing in terms of material assistance. Therefore for the purposes of clarity it is important to separate conceptually these differing forms of familialism.

Workforce reform

The 2004 Children Act promises a 'workforce reform strategy', the purpose of which will be to increase the effectiveness, skills, training, retention and recruitment of the 'children's workforce'. No one could reasonably object to better training and a better career structure aimed at recruiting and retaining social workers, and others who work with children and their families, who face the daunting task of supporting children and their families whilst simultaneously policing and detecting child abuse, especially given the tragic consequences which sometimes happen and which form the central focus of this book.

However, having freely acknowledged this, there are two important things to bear in mind about it. First, it should be remembered that there is a strong tradition within the British state of responding to perceived crises in public issues of childcare by setting up public inquiries, which often call for increased training for social workers. Second, they often also call for increased knowledge and more research. For instance, the Home Office Children's Committee was set up as a result of the death of a child in a nautical training school in 1910. The Curtis Committee of 1945 was set up as a result of the death of a child in foster care, and it recommended a specific training qualification in childcare. Many subsequent shifts in policy, research and training are responses to public childcare tragedies. Hence, there remains a risk of producing simply another incremental dose of the sorts of discourses and ideologies outlined and critiqued earlier since, quite apart from anything else, this book argues that a central problem which assists in producing unintended and tragic consequences is the way in which the statutory duties of social workers have been framed over time, and are still currently framed.

Corby (2006) in his comprehensive review of the current 'knowledge base' in relation to child abuse points out that any reasonable approach to the problem, needs at least an ability to describe its nature and its size, in order that the response to it may be appropriately resourced and therefore effectively tackled. However, he adds that

> the notions of child abuse and neglect are complex, subject to constant change and realignment. They are highly contested concepts, underpinned by and subject to a range of political and cultural factors particular to the society in which they occur. For these reasons child abuse and neglect are not phenomena that lend themselves to easy definition or measurement.
>
> (p. 79)

There is nevertheless much to be learned from competing perspectives and differing attempts to research and conceptualise the problem, though in such circumstances there will always be a problem for the practitioner, in the here and now, of evaluating and applying to specific individual cases, competing evidence and knowledge, even where it can all be successfully absorbed. This is no simple matter for the very busy practitioner.

In this endeavour, the development of 'evidence-based practice' can be of genuine assistance to such social workers on the ground, but it should not be assumed that acquiring skills in this area is a simple matter, as Macdonald (2001), in a book dedicated to developing evidence-based practice, points out

> Child protection is a complex social endeavour. It is one of the few areas where the state seeks to intervene in an otherwise private

arena, that of family life, and where a range of professional groups and organizations, as well as the general public, are expected to play a part. It is a problematic endeavour too. Child physical abuse, child neglect, psychological maltreatment and child sexual abuse are all socially constructed in ways which make definition, discussion and decision making technically challenging.

(p. xvii)

There is no seamless glide between a concern to tackle the serious problem of child abuse in all of its forms and a skilled evidence-based, historically informed, effective social-work practice in relation to it, though of course this does not mean that such endeavours should not be fully supported and funded.

The definitions of abuse that are currently operational in social-work practice are essentially formal ones, for instance, the 'threshold criteria' of 'significant harm' originally established the 1989 Act which must be crossed to justify statutory intervention. Setting aside the fact that there is 'no absolute criteria on which to rely when judging what constitutes significant harm' (Department of Health, Home Office, Department of Education and Employment 1999: 7), it needs to be remembered that much that we might genuinely consider to be inappropriate care, if not actually child abuse, takes place prior to this threshold being reached. This begs the very question with which this book is engaged, that is, the tension between support for children and their families and caretakers on the one hand and statutory intervention on the other. This difficulty is recognised in a relatively recent government funded research study (Department of Health 2001), which reports that

> Simultaneous safeguarding and promoting children's welfare has been difficult to achieve. It is clear that, on the one hand, some children have not been made the subject of care proceedings soon enough. In other cases, the operation of a high threshold for family support has led to insufficient intervention at an early stage.

(p. 143)

The Department of Health in their *Working Together to Safeguard Children* (1999) offer formal definitions of physical abuse, emotional abuse, sexual abuse and neglect and it is often these definitions, linked with the legal threshold of 'significant harm' which inform policy and practice on the ground. Useful as these are to the practitioner, the guidance nevertheless points out that

> Judgements on how best to intervene when there are concerns about harm to a child will often and unavoidably entail an element of risk – at the extreme, of leaving a child for too long in a dangerous situation or of removing a child unnecessarily from their family.
>
> (p. 2)

The guidance deals with this uncertainty by suggesting that what is required is 'competent professional judgments based on sound assessment of the child's needs', together with an assessment of the parents' ability to meet those needs – 'including their capacity to keep the child from significant harm – and the wider family circumstances' (p. 2). A tough job – especially when situations vary and are unclear. In her Introduction, for example, to the Department of Health's 2002 *Learning from Past Experience: A Review of Serious Case Reviews* (Sinclair and Bullock 2002), the then Minster of State for Community, Jacqui Smith, pointed out that

> In some cases, the abuse occurred out of the blue, in others it occurred in a context of low level need and occasionally it arose in situations where it seemed to have been 'waiting to happen'.
>
> (p. i)

Clearly, in practice, this level of uncertainty adds to the difficulties that social workers face, and in many ways it is a testimony to their skill and humanity 'on the ground' that there are not many more tragedies on their caseloads.

The assessment of these risks has been the subject of much practical attention in recent years and the *Framework for the Assessment of Children in Need and their Families* ((Department of Health 2000), now being supplemented by the new 2005 *Common Assessment Framework for Children and Young People* (Department of Health 2005) are of assistance. But the guidance to the latter points out that 'resources are finite' and simply doing a common assessment

> cannot guarantee that services (especially those involving another agency) will be delivered. However, agencies should agree their priorities locally so as to maximize the outcomes for children and minimize the risk that identified needs will not receive an adequate response.
>
> (p. 4)

It is issues such as those considered above that lead to the recognition of the limits of what can be achieved by enhanced knowledge and training. Both of these things are of course to be warmly welcomed, since they may well produce social workers who are better able to cope with these contradictions, and even negotiate them, but the central dilemma within child-protection system remains unresolved, even if it is at times recognised and acknowledged. If the 2004 Act provides no radical rethink of the problem of child protection, and this book suggests that is so, and also attempts to illustrate why it is so, (i.e. in significant measure because of conflicting statutory duties laid upon social service departments, and their successors, effectively in the personage of the social worker on the ground and his or her supervisors and managers in the 1989 Act), then there is no good reason to suppose, though of course we all may hope, that childcare tragedies will not continue to happen.

A separation of functions?

Considerations such as those outlined immediately above, and throughout this book, may lead to a temptation to advocate the separating of the investigation and detection of child abuse, that is, the elements within childcare law which are connected with the discourse of punishment, from the prevention and treatment of child abuse and the rehabilitation of children within once abusing families/households. However, this may be, in the end, easier said than done. After all, workers on the ground, often find themselves involved in a corrosive continuum of neglectful childcare which only sometimes shades into a level of abuse which crosses the legal threshold of significant harm.

If, for instance, all investigation were undertaken by the police (by specially trained investigative workers) then this in itself might, whatever its intention, appear to people, children included, as heavy-handed and therefore produce a lack of cooperation arising from fear of prosecution or parental reprisal. There is the problem that not all that might be considered abuse would be of a criminal nature and not all investigations lead to prosecution, or even registration. There would therefore be not only be the problem of the location of an appropriate threshold of intervention, there would also be the problem of the thresholds involved in transferring cases between the police and social workers and, sometimes, back again. In addition there would be the issue of training for the police officers involved and the resource implications of devoting more police time to this issue. In any event there is little evidence to suggest that the police would welcome this addition to their role.

It might be suggested instead that different teams of specially trained social workers, as currently in certain children and family teams, who only undertake child-protection work, should fulfil these differing roles and functions. Many of the problems outlined above would still remain (e.g. the thresholds at which different teams become involved and re-involved in any particular case). This would require reorganisation and significantly increased resources. All of this focuses essentially, in one way or another, on the institutional management of the problem (Sinclair and Corden 2005), and not on policies designed to reduce the incidence of the problem.

In addition to the above, there are therefore issues of 'wider social change', for example, greater levels of economic and social and physical support for parents/caretakers, families, households and children such as increased childcare benefits, increased levels of preschool education, the granting of greater rights and autonomy to children, the tackling of the question of child poverty and increased employment and education opportunities for the members of the society in which we live. In more global terms, more humane treatment for asylum-seeking children and their families, and more reluctance to resort to war, with all the appalling consequences for children that is its inevitable consequence, are both important. Without a commitment to wider social change, institutional policy changes will run the risk of simply becoming another incremental policy shift along the same trajectory, in a long line of such discursively and ideologically produced shifts of policy emphasis.

Children's rights

It is for this reason that I suggest in Chapter 3 that the government in not acting upon its obligation to implement United Nations Convention on the Rights of the Child, has declined an important opportunity to raise the social and economic status of children and young people by giving them a firmer voice in all matters that impact upon them. However, in the 2004 Children Act, the UK government focused, instead of this, on the five broad outcomes goals outlined in *Every Child Matters*. Had they instead focused upon a plan of action on the implementation of the Convention they would have potentially produced far stronger child-protection measures. It is worth restating that, article 12 of the Convention says,

> 1   States Parties shall assure to the child who is capable of forming his or her own views the right to express those views freely in all matters affecting the child, the views of the child being given due weight in accordance with the age and maturity of the child.

2   For this purpose, the child shall in particular be provided the opportunity to be heard in any judicial and administrative proceedings affecting the child, either directly, or through a representative or an appropriate body, in a manner consistent with the procedural rules of national law.

Clearly, this places an obligation on all concerned with direct work with children to fully engage with them. This centralises the rights of the child within child protection, and indeed in regard to all other matters that impact upon them. It is surely worth recollecting, in relation to the tragic story of Victoria Climbié, that, as discussed earlier, Victoria was known to three housing authorities, four social services departments, two child-protection teams of the Metropolitan Police Service, a specialist centre managed by the NSPCC, and two different hospitals.

A social-work practice that was driven by the human rights of Victoria, under the UN Convention, in particular article 12, might have avoided this tragic outcome, if only for the simple reason that it would require a direct one to one engagement with her by all with whom her family came into professional contact. Sadly, it would appear that such a level of engagement was missing in this tragic case, and this, independently of any particular organisational arrangements, might have saved her life (though of course, distressing mistakes are a sad part of the human condition, especially in the enormously difficult and highly complex field of child abuse).

A children's rights 'driver' in child-protection practice would require a change in the social context in which issues of child abuse and neglect are seen, identified, dealt with, and in some in significant measure, even constructed. It would involve the recognition of children and young people as citizens in their own right, and not simply and solely as the 'property' of their parents and caretakers. Granting children and young people the same status and voice as adults within the child-protection system is still some way off, especially in relation to younger children, or children who do not communicate verbally, even though techniques exist to facilitate communication with such children.

An example of societal ambivalence in relation to the issue of children's rights is the fact that it remains legal to physically punish children under s.58 of the Children Act 2004 providing that there are no injuries that would justify an assault charge. Perhaps the question could be posed as to whether the law would remain framed in this way, if under article 12 of the UN Convention, children and young people were asked what their views were about such a law.

I hope this book makes a small contribution towards facilitating a recognition of the particular problem with which it is concerned, if it focuses social workers, social-work educators and policy makers on the problems which are rooted in the way in which the task of childcare intervention has been constructed legislatively over time, we may hope for a greater understanding of the very real difficulties social workers face in the here-and-now in carrying out that task. This in turn may lead to more sympathetic and humane responses to workers who face the personal and professional agony of a child abuse tragedy on their caseload. I hope too it may lead to a deeper commitment to engaging directly with children and young people in both in child-protection policy and practice.

A counter-discourse

In a discussion with Giles Deleuze first published in a special issue of L'Arc which was dedicated to Giles Deleuze, Michel Foucault, speaking of his work with the 'Groupe d'information des prisons' suggests that

> In the most recent upheaval [he is referring to the events of May 1968 in Paris], the intellectual discovered that the masses no longer need him to gain knowledge, they *know* perfectly well, without illusion, they know far better than he and they are certainly capable of expressing themselves. But there exists a system of power which blocks, prohibits, and invalidates this discourse and this knowledge...

He later adds

> And when the prisoners began to speak, they possessed an individual theory of prisons, the penal system, and justice. It is this form of discourse which ultimately matters, a discourse against power, the counter-discourse of prisoners and those we call delinquents – and not a theory about delinquency.
>
> (Foucault 1972)

As a part of the initial research for this book, and in the above spirit, I wished to obtain some young people's perceptions of the public-care system, based upon their experience of it. I felt that the subjects/objects of powerful discourses should be permitted to speak for themselves. I felt that it was important that their counter-discourse be heard.

I was nevertheless anxious about the best way to do this. Clearly there were issues of power involved in interviewing very young people on a one-to-one basis. I felt that the young people might feel more empowered to speak if (a) they were in a group, (b) they were on their own territory and (c) they were in the older age range, for example, 16 years plus. This latter point would also help in the sense that young people of this age might have had some years of involvement with the system and have more to offer, but also may have had more time to make their own sense of the experience. Bearing all these factors in mind I facilitated a group interview and discussion. The names of the young people concerned have been changed in order to protect their anonymity, as has the name of the social services department with which they were involved.

Anytown Social Services Department, who kindly gave permission for this interview, providing of course they remain anonymous, have a resource, the purpose of which is to offer bed-sit accommodation to young people who have been in their care, which they rent and within which they provide their own food and do their own cooking etc.

In discussing my work with the worker in charge of this resource, she suggested that she could put up a notice inviting anyone who wished to meet me and discuss their experiences of the care system. She also knew of a number of people who had recently moved on whom she thought might be interested in joining such a discussion, and she agreed to contact them and invite them on the date agreed.

The appendix that follows is a transcription of the discussions that took place between the young people and myself. I *feel that it is important not to offer an analysis of this transcript.* I believe that to do so would be to risk recapturing the counter-discourse of the young people and mobilising it as a part of my own discourse. This would of course be contrary to the concept and spirit of counter-discourse as outlined earlier.

On the evening concerned there were, at various times, up to 10 young people in the room. They varied in age from 16 to 22 years. There was also a small party taking place to say goodbye to the member of staff in question. Before commencing I clarified with the young people whether they wished to use some of their evening in this way and whether they minded, given an undertaking of confidentiality, if the discussion was taped to be subsequently used as part of my research. I was surprised that they responded very enthusiastically to the idea, suggesting that the music be turned off, the tape recorder placed on the table, and we would 'see what happened next'. What happened next was that these young people spoke volumes on their own behalf. Hence I feel the final discourse that a reader of this book should consider is that of the young people concerned and this is why it is included as an appendix.

Appendix

A counter-discourse involving a number of young people who had either recently left care or were still in care at the time

The discussion begins with a young man who describes the system as 'total shit'. Many of the young people seem to have had bad experiences in one particular children's home – the rules are too rigidly applied and they are changed regularly without consultation. The young man is particularly angered by this, though perhaps there are elements of his playing to an audience. This was confirmed by a young woman who later said, 'In my home they would take advantage of people who couldn't stand up for themselves – like [the young man in question] for Instance – he's making out he's something that he's not, now he's more louder, but then they dominated him.'

D.M.: Who dominated him, the kids or the staff?

YOUNG WOMAN: Staff, not the kids, we were all together, you see. If anything happened we'd say can you say this, you can say that. If they could get away with it they did you know – but they couldn't like with me or... – they didn't. You know, you get a clothing allowance every month, well, I didn't come in one night – it was a real emergency actually – my sister was ill and I went to see her, and they didn't believe me. They stopped my clothing allowance for a year, a whole year!

D.M.: A year?

YOUNG WOMAN: Yes, a whole year. At the end of the year they gave it back to me all at once because they had to.

D.M.: 'Cos of just one night? You must have been furious!

YOUNG WOMAN: I made out I didn't care. I did care. My social worker wouldn't do nothing.

The conversation turns to another Anytown home. A young man says that it is good because in there you are 'under manners'. A young woman contradicts, 'If you only do things 'cos if you don't your pocket money gets stopped, it's not real, is it?'

YOUNG WOMAN: That's different but like, say, it's something very minor – like forgetting to do your laundry – you got fined. When you came home you had to polish your shoes straight away. People didn't do that, right? They were tired, they'd go upstairs and have a shower first and they'd stop your pocket money, and that would be for weeks on end. If you're not down for supper by half past eight you miss or you lose your pocket money.

ANOTHER YOUNG WOMAN: My brother was there and what did he have? A wardrobe and a mattress on the floor – that was it!

YOUNG MAN: You should have nicked a bed.

YOUNG WOMAN: You couldn't find one to nick.

A young man approached me, wanting to be in a more one-to-one situation, and told me that his experiences were good, though he had been in a lot of homes. He added, 'I went back to live with my mother for 2 months. In the end my dad clamped down on that. I went somewhere else but I started getting problems with the residents. I walked out... on and off I kept getting into fights.... I left and after that I came here.'

D.M.: That guy who's gone said if you weren't under manners things would be over the top. Is that right?

YOUNG WOMAN: No, it's not!

ANOTHER YOUNG WOMAN: I'm not agreeing with what they did to you, right? But taking away your pocket money is a way of putting you under manners. But they took it too far with you lot. See what I mean? Children's homes have the right as well as parents.

D.M.: What makes a place nice?

YOUNG WOMAN: The staff. They shouldn't be allowed to do the job unless they like kids and really want to do it.

YOUNG WOMAN: It's not only that. They have this attitude, 'I'm a social worker. I'm trained in this field. I know what you are feeling. I am always going to be right. You can't tell me nothing. If you're crying and your friend comes up to you, well, your friend can't help you. I can help you.'

OTHER YOUNG WOMAN: But you don't know. You've got to live it, and you shouldn't be allowed to do it unless you actually like kids. A degree in psychology's not it.

D.M. summarises some of the issues that have been raised and asks if there is anything positive that the young people could say about the system, a particular experience, a particular social worker or particular key worker, perhaps? There was some laughter and a young man said 'dig deep'. D.M. said, 'Well, OK then, the other way – anything really stupid that you just wouldn't credit could happen?'

YOUNG WOMAN: I went into a children's home and they didn't have any Afro combs. They gave me a little nit comb, right?

ANOTHER YOUNG WOMAN: We used to get five pounds a month toiletries. How are you supposed to clean your skin? I'm lucky I don't have afro hair or nothing, right? I'm talking on behalf of the other black people there. How are you supposed to grease your hair? How are you supposed to keep your skin clean? We had to fight, fight, fight for more money. Even though there were three black workers there you still had to fight for it.

YOUNG WOMAN: They see everyone as white, you know, all the same. Why should anybody be treated differently? But you *are* different.

D.M.: Did you get support from the black workers there?

YOUNG WOMAN: Well, yeah, after a while, because I was having to use my hairdressing money. Everyone is given the same hairdressing money, aren't they? But it costs more to get your hair done if you're black, and another thing is food. I was in care for a year, right, and I went mad. If you are black or Asian you don't eat. You wake up in the morning and it's bacon and eggs: I don't eat bacon and eggs. I don't eat pork. They don't cater for people's religions, stuff like that. I mean, bangers and mash – as if anybody is going to sit down and eat that, and you say, 'What's this?' and they say, 'It's dinner', and you think, 'If I was at home it would be rice and peas' – know what I mean?

YOUNG WOMAN: Some of the staff don't understand the person that you are. All the anger that's inside you, stopping your pocket money and things – you turn round and say: 'You wouldn't treat your own kids like that – you wouldn't lock up the TV room' if you've got a lot of anger inside you. I know I was like that when I was younger. I've changed since then. I didn't know what I was angry for. It's only in the past two years that I have been learning about my life – it fucks you up, it really does.

D.M.: I understand what you mean.

SAME YOUNG WOMAN: When I was with foster parents for 10 years and it broke down I thought I was a failure, but I didn't know what I was doing wrong. My parents gave me up when I was 3 months old, my foster parents when I was two. I've been in care for the rest of my life, it's hard to explain it...I don't know.

D.M.: What I understand from what you're saying – correct me if I'm wrong – is that you had a lot of anger inside you and a lot of bad feelings inside you which you are only just beginning to work out, but that actually locking up the television room doesn't much help. It doesn't make you any less angry, does it?

YOUNG WOMAN: That's right. You don't realise what you're angry about. You can't express it without lashing out or whatever. They used to provoke you more, you know.

D.M.: So pointless rules and food that you don't like just winds you up?

YOUNG WOMAN: They don't know how to cope with your anger. I went into care from home, right? I thought home was heaven compared to being in care, but they didn't understand that. The first time I was in tears, I was nearly hysterical, and I asked them to let me use the phone. They let me call Watford for hours, because the staff there didn't know how to cope with me.

D.M.: Because they weren't able to just sit down with you?

YOUNG WOMAN: They don't know when to sit down with you or when to leave you alone.

D.M.: I honestly don't want to take up all your evening. We can stop if you like?

YOUNG MAN: I've got quite a lot out of this evening. So has anybody ever been better off in a home?

YOUNG WOMAN: It depends how you look at it. When you're at home you're thinking, 'Oh God, let me get out of this.' As soon as you get into care you're thinking, 'I'm going to leave now.' I know what you were saying about...because my brother was there sleeping on a mattress on the floor, and you said, 'Nick a bed from another room.' You couldn't find a bed to nick, you couldn't find a bed to nick, *you couldn't find a bed to nick – right?*

YOUNG MAN: When was he there?

YOUNG WOMAN: He was there about 4 years ago.

(The young people all felt that this place had gone down hill. There was a discussion about locking up the food cupboard which contained mouldy bread.)

D.M.: You said that sometimes, for some reason, OK, you didn't want to be at home and, alright, when you went into care that was no good either, they locked up mouldy bread! Was there anything else that could have helped – other places? Crash pads? Anything at all?

YOUNG WOMAN: A little more understanding. You check it, right, check it like this. When my brother was there he was 16 and he used to go out and do a couple of yards and things, right, and then go back. Now at the age of 16 you need your freedom, and then again you need to be checked – I'm sorry if that offends anyone but you need to be checked too. That just completely freaked him out because he thought, 'If I was at home I wouldn't be able to get away with this anyway' – know what I mean?

YOUNG WOMAN: I'm going now but I want to say one thing, right? There is a lot of bad staff in children's homes, but you've got to give credit to the good ones. When I was at the … I really, really hated it, but there were some good staff.

D.M.: And they were really important to you, were they?

YOUNG WOMAN: They were really important and there should be more – then it would be nicer in homes.

(At this point some young people leave – there are 'bye 'bye's, etc.)

D.M.: I think we should stop and get on with your leaving party.

YOUNG MAN: No, not really.

(We do another round of names.)

I was asked had I been in care myself – I explained that I hadn't but that I had worked in a home. I explained my present job – and the reason I was doing the research – I said I wanted to get student social workers to listen to and read about what young people said about the system.

A young person asked me what I thought of what I had heard so far. I said that I felt that I already knew some of the things that they had told me but that it really mattered that *they* were saying them. All this took place against a backcloth of general conversation. A young woman asked what to do about a superintendent who was doing bad stuff to the kids – the issue was physical violence – we discussed how you had to go about proving something like that, witness, adults you can trust, etc. The young woman talked about a situation where this was happening and the social worker challenged it and it was denied and matters were left at that. She said, 'It sickens me that he has got promoted – he shouldn't have that position. He shouldn't be a social worker, full stop. Never mind telling other social workers to do this or that.'

We discussed this further and I gave what advice I could at a general level about how to go about dealing with a situation like that. I suggested that she discuss it with the member of staff who had arranged the evening and whom she trusts; she agreed to do so. I also mentioned the conversation to the worker at a later time.

YOUNG MAN: When I came into care I had no clothes, my mother spent all her money, the only way I could get clothes was to nick them; at least when I came into care I got clothes.

YOUNG WOMAN: I've been in a lot of children's homes since I was 13. I've been in care since I was three. I can forget all the slaps, all the beatings for ridiculous things. I remember being sent down the shop for a bar of chocolate and when I came back, being a child I hid it. He asked Jenny ... where it was, and she didn't know. He slapped her and kicked her all round the room. He came to me and I said I hid it. It didn't occur to him to even say sorry to Jenny. ... (She continues) Alright, I can forget all that but for *all those years* the only thing – I mean you can have money and clothes. I mean everybody knows you have fashionable clothes when you're in care – older care. I mean when I was younger I used to get the rejects from other children's homes around me.... The only time you ever get *touched* is if you are crying, or if you try to commit suicide. It's the only time you ever have any contact and that's why most of the girls, when they get to be 14, 15, they sleep with the *first man* when they come along because it is the first bit of contact that you would have got in years, and that is the saddest, saddest thing about being in care. You see all these young girls going to bed with every Tom, Dick or Harry because the only contact they have had in their lives is when they have gone to bed with somebody, and it is sad. I've done it, I know I've done it, and I know hundreds of other girls who have done it.... I can remember precisely, it was on my fourteenth birthday that I got a kiss on the cheek, and that was the first piece of contact I had in God knows how long, and that was because I was 14 and becoming a big girl, and that was from a woman. You just get to the stage where you want to cringe if someone wants to touch you. Leave me alone, because it feels just so uncomfortable for someone to put their arms around you.

D.M.: Because you're denied physical contact?

YOUNG WOMAN: Yeah, because you don't want it and 'Leave me alone, I'm hard.' You don't need that shit. I know loads of people in here that have done it.

ANOTHER YOUNG WOMAN: When you go on the street you have to act hard because you are in care and that's what's expected of you.

A THIRD YOUNG WOMAN: You have to be a bit hard if you are in care. You can't be stupid and let everyone walk all over you.

FIRST YOUNG WOMAN: You take a young, naive child and you put them in care. You really have to be careful about what home you put them in to depend on which way their life is going to go. I've seen really nice people go into one home or another and at the end of it's turned out a right fucking – it's just fucked them up completely.

D.M.: Was it all around Anytown?

YOUNG WOMAN: No, my sister, she was fostered, and I went from this to that to this to that, like the biggest parts of my life were spent in . . . , then I went home for 3 years, well 2 years, from when I was 11 to 13, then I lived in . . . . I lived there twice, those are the bigger parts of my life, the bits I remember. I've read my file and I know the other bits – that's why files are important – but yes, they should be kept away from everybody else's eyes. I'd never know how many social workers I've had – I could never count them – moving from home to home to home. You can never expect to trust anybody – because the next week you might not be there – the next day another staff comes on. I think, 'This is crazy, how can I stand here and talk to you when I might not be here next week, or when you might tell everybody.' That's the difficult thing – they should take more time. I mean, these are people's lives, aren't they?

D.M.: How did you survive it, if that's not too personal a question?

YOUNG WOMAN: I'll tell you what you do. You build a fortress around yourself so much that at the end of it you feel that you are incapable of love or care, because it's just you you have to look after. For so long I believed that I could never love anybody, like anybody. I mean inside I was the softest thing, I was so lost. (She continues) You would never believe it if I sat in front of you 4 years ago, you would think just look at this shitty little girl, 'cos I was. I was abusive, I'd spit at you, I'd kick at you, I'd scream at you. I'd do anything and that's why now, when I see kids like that I could never, never, never think, 'Oh, little shit!' 'or little this' or 'little that'. I just think: 'Shit, they must just be so fucking lonely, they must be hurting so much to be like that.' (She adds) . . . Because I have no friends – I never had any. They were all scared of me – that's why they wanted to *be* my friends – know what I mean? I never had any *real* friends. And then getting out of that is more difficult than getting in it, much more – to try and learn to like and care about people, even though you do – to *show it*.

D.M.: Because you get into it bit by bit – do you? I mean just from day to day, keeping people away from you?

YOUNG WOMAN: For a lot, a lot, a lot of years. I mean the only person who would try and comfort me was my mum, for a lot of years I would literally think I was going to vomit if she kissed me. If she put her arms round me I wouldn't like it. It's only been in the last couple of years that I can cuddle her. I mean I know it's not her fault. I can't blame anybody for what's happened, it's just you do that to yourself. It's the care system that does it. You shove a whole lot of poor kids into one children's home and you treat them like they are all exactly the same – like they haven't got their own Individual problems. Just give them the same old food – whether they're Turkish, Greek, black or whatever; it doesn't matter. I mean . . . half Chinese and they stuck her out in the middle of bloody [a rural county]. She was the only Chinese person there. She doesn't know anything about her own culture and I don't because my father is Turkish. I don't know anything about my own culture – anything about anything. I'm English now and nothing can change it. My father's Turkish and my mother's Irish. You just lose your culture – you are supposed to just regain that after you leave. I wish . . . would talk because she has so much to say. God knows, I've sat up until five o'clock in the morning listening to it. She should talk.

THE YOUNG WOMAN IN QUESTION: That's a strong point with me, black people in care, because I went to college for 2 years and I did a whole project on black and in care. I went out with questionnaires. It's a strong point with me, black people in care – especially mixed. I'm mixed, you see, my mother is white and my father is black and when you are in care you get a bit mixed up, it's confusing.

D.M.: Because you're made Invisible?

ANGELA: Yeah. I'm seen as black because my skin is black.

D.M.: Where were you in care – in Anytown?

ANGELA: All over. I started in . . . then I was in . . . I've been in care all my life. Then I went out to . . . – to the countryside – with nuns, and then I came back to . . . to live here.

D.M.: How long did you live with nuns?

ANGELA: About 2 years.

D.M.: That must have been weird?

ANGELA: There were only about three of us and they didn't have a clue how to look after us anyway, they just shut us in our room.

D.M.: They shut you in your room?

ANGELA: Yeah. If they couldn't cope with us they'd shut us in our room. That's how they worked.

D.M.: (after a pause) When did you realise that your identity was being denied?

ANGELA: After I left. I went to college and did a social care course and they did a lot on racism.

ANOTHER YOUNG (BLACK) WOMAN: Does the term half-caste offend *you*?

ANGELA: Yeah. I prefer mixed race.

ANOTHER YOUNG WOMAN: They don't understand your needs because they don't know whether you as an Individual want to take one side or the other, or whether you just want to take the mainstream. Like anybody has the right to take whatever identify they choose, but there is a secret little code that is unspoken that once you are a certain colour you must take a certain culture, and you must stick to that because that *is your culture.*

YOUNG WOMAN: One thing I want to say is that as soon as you are in care and you're black they think, oh, troublemaker, let's bung 'em up somewhere – criminal. I've been pulled up often for no obvious reason.

YOUNG MAN: I get pulled all the time and I'm not black.

ANOTHER YOUNG MAN: Yeah, but you *look like a criminal.*

A YOUNG WOMAN: Can you tell me why they split people up who are related? I've got two sisters, one is black, the other white, same mother, different dads, right? And from the time we were in care from eight, we were always split up – for no reason at all. Up to now I still don't know. I was in... another sister was in... not a mile and a half away and my other sister was up in..., and she was fostered – she must have agreed to that – you have to, don't you? I used to spend weekends and go on holiday together and, if I was lucky, once or twice in the week, but they would never let us live together, and my other sister Debbie is about 4 years older than me and they would never let us live together, and I know lots of other kids like that.

ANOTHER YOUNG WOMAN: *My* brother was put in the... and I was put with foster parents.

FIRST YOUNG WOMAN: Perhaps they think that they don't want you together. It will make things hard. I don't know?

D.M.: Well, what do you think about that?

YOUNG WOMAN: They just stick you anywhere there is space. But you want to be with people you have spent some part of your life with. 'Cos we just came from Wales and we didn't know nothing at all.

D.M.: And they split you up?

YOUNG WOMAN: Yeah. For maybe a year, and then she ran away and then I went.

D.M.: Did they never tell you why you were split up? Did you never ask?

YOUNG WOMAN: If I was depressed I'd go and see her, and they would let us spend the night – one superintendent would ring the other and say, 'I'll make sure she goes to school.' I'd get a ride in the van.

D.M.: That must have felt really strange for you. Just being split up and not knowing why?

ANOTHER YOUNG WOMAN: I have two sisters – they put me in... and my sister in..., it was miles and miles and miles away and the hardest thing was I couldn't get to see them. I used to see her about twice a year. I used to have to go to my social worker and say, 'I want to see....' Then they would have a meeting, then they would have a meeting with Susan's social worker and then a meeting to make up the date. We're not even like sisters. I hardly even know her. I love her because she is my sister. So they ripped a whole family apart. It's sick, isn't it?

D.M.: Yes, it's sick.

YOUNG WOMAN: Because they don't give a fuck. They can't give a fuck if they do that. They don't even give you the proper access to develop a relationship over the years and so now all of a sudden my sister is 18 and now I can see my sister. Well, thank you very much! I mean that's what I had to wait for, until she was big enough that she was going to live near me, when I started to realise, when I got to 16, they said, 'Right, you can go and see her', and it was me that had to do all the work, and then it was even still more difficult. Well, I've got a big sister in name, but I mean I hardly see this woman – know what I mean? She might be my sister in name but that's about it. Then from then, from an older age you have to build a relationship and that is so hard, a relationship between two women – like friends only you have the same blood. It's sick. They need shooting, those people, I think we should all do it, what do you reckon? Stand them all up against the wall.

A YOUNG WOMAN: I want to say one more thing. I had a bad time in a children's home, but if I hadn't been there I wouldn't be here. I might not have got my flat, and I might have had nowhere to live. So there's one good point. The rest is shit, for me, personally, that's it.

FIRST YOUNG WOMAN: I'd never be as strong as I am now if I hadn't gone through it. If I'd have stayed with my mum I would be chaos. I reckon more kids in care should become social workers.

YOUNG MAN: Yeah! They'd make good social workers, they would.

The group of young people felt that it was time to return to their party. I thanked them very warmly for their time. A young man turned on the radio and the reggae programme played a request from the young people dedicated to the worker who had arranged the discussion, and who was leaving.

Bibliography

Addison, P. (1975) *The Road to 1945*, Jonathan Cape.

Althusser, L. (1971) *Lenin and Philosophy*, Monthly Review Press.

Ashenden, A. (1990) 'Habermas' theory of communicative action: an analysis of the thesis of the "Internal Colonization of the Lifeworld"', unpublished doctoral thesis.

Assiter, A. (2003) *Revisiting Universalism*, Palgrave, Macmillan.

Bailey, M. and Brake, R. (eds) (1975) *Radical Social Work*, Arnold.

—— (1980) *Radical Social Work and Practice*, Arnold.

Bolger, S., Corrigan, P., Docking, J. and Frost, N. (1981) *Towards Socialist Welfare Work*, Macmillan.

Bowlby, J. (1978) *Attachment*, Penguin Books.

Brill, K. (1976) 'Preface' in Leeding, A. (ed.) *A Child Care Manual for Social Workers*, Butterworth.

Callinicos, A. (1989) *Against Postmodernism – A Marxist Critique*, Polity Press.

Callinicos, A. and Harman, C. (1987) *The Changing Working Class*, Bookmarks.

Chibnall, S. (1977) *Law and Order News: An Analysis of Crime in the British Press*. Tauistock.

Children's Rights Alliance of England (2005) *State of Children's Rights in England 2005 – Annual review of the UK Government Action on 2002 Concluding Observations of the United Nations Committee on the Rights of the Child*, Children's Rights Alliance for England.

Clarke, J. (1985) 'Managing the delinquent: the children's branch of the Home Office 1913–1930', in Langan, M. and Schwarz, B. (eds) *Crisis in the British State. 1880–1930*, Hutchinson.

Clarke, J., Gewirtz, S. and McLaughlin, E. (eds) (2000) *New Managerialism, New Welfare*, Sage.

Cleveland County Council (1988) *Report of the Inquiry into Child Abuse in Cleveland 1987 – Short Version Extracted from the Complete Text*, DHSS/HMSO.

Cohen, S. (1973) *Folk Devils and Moral Panics*, Paladin.

Corby, B. (2006) *Child Abuse – Towards a Knowledge Base*, Open University Press.

Corrigan, P. and Leonard, E. (1981) *Social Work Practice Under Capitalism*, Macmillan.

Curtis Committee (1946a) *The Report of the Interdepartmental Committee on Training and Child Care (The Interim Report of the Curtis Committee)*, Cmnd 6760, HMSO.

—— (1946b) *Report of the Interdepartmental Committee on the Care of Children (The Curtis Report)*, Cmnd 6922, HMSO.

David, M. (1991) 'Putting on an act for children', in Maclean, M. and Groves, D. (eds) *Women's Issues in Social Policy*, Routledge.

Department of Education and Skills (2005) *Common Assessment Framework for Children and Young People – Guide for Service Managers and Practitioners*, Department for Education and Skills.

Department of Health (1991) *Working Together – Under the Children Act: A Guide to Inter-agency Co-operation for the Protection of Children from Abuse*, HMSO.

—— (2000) *Framework for the Assessment of Children in Need and their Families*, The Stationery Office.

—— (2001) *The Children Act Now – Messages from Research*, The Stationery Office.

—— (2003) *Every Child Matters*, Cmnd 5860, The Stationery Office.

Department of Health, Home Office, Department for Education and Employment (1999) *Working Together to Safeguard Children*, The Stationery Office.

DHSS (1974) *Report of the Committee of Inquiry into the Care and Supervision Provided in Relation to Maria Colwell*, HMSO.

—— (1985) *Review of Child Care Law – Report to Ministers of an Interdepartmental Working Party*, HMSO.

Dominelli, L. (1988) *Anti-Racist Social Work*, Macmillan.

Dominelli, L. and McCleod, E. (1989) *Feminist Social Work*, Macmillan.

Dreyfus, H. L. and Rabinow, P. (1982) *Michel Foucault – Beyond Structuralism and Hermeneutics*, Harvester.

DSS (1995) *Child Protection – The Messages From Research*, HMSO.

Eagleton, T. (1991) *Ideology – An Introduction*, Verso.

Elliot, P. (1972) *Sociology of Professions*, Macmillan.

Fairclough, N. (1989) *Language and Power*, Longman.

Finkelhor, D. (ed.) (1986) *A Sourcebook on Child Sexual Abuse*, Sage.

Ford, D. (1975) *Children, Courts and Caring: A Study of the Children and Young Persons Act 1969*, Constable Publications.

Foucault, M. (1965) *Madness and Civilization: A History of Insanity in the Age of Reason*. Translated by Richard Howard. Pantheon.

—— (1972) 'Intellectuals and power', *L'Arc*, 495: 3–10.

—— (1977) 'The political function of the intellectual', *Radical Philosophy*, 17 (Summer): 12–14.

—— (1978) 'Politics and the study of discourse', *Ideology and Consciousness*, 3: 7–26.

—— (1980) in Gibson, C. (ed.) *Power/Knowledge*, Harvester.

—— (1981) 'Questions of method: an interview with Michel Foucault', *Ideology and Consciousness*, 8: 3–14.

—— (1982) 'The subject and power – afterword', in Dreyfus, H. L. and Rabinow, P. (eds) *Michel Foucault – Beyond Structuralism and Hermeneutics*, Harvester.

—— (1984) *The History of Sexuality*, Peregrine Books.

—— (1986) 'Nietzsche, genealogy, history', in Rabinow, P. (ed.) *The Foucault Reader*, Peregrine Books.

Fox Harding, L. (1991) *Perspectives in Child Care Policy,* Longman.

Freeman, M. (1993) 'Laws, conventions and rights', *Children and Society*, 7: 1, 37–48.

Frost, N. and Stein, M. (1989) *The Politics of Child Welfare – Inequality, Power and Change*, Harvester Wheatsheaf.

Geras, N. (1983) *Marx and Human Nature, Refutation of a Legend*, Verso Editions and NLB.

Gilroy, P. (1987) *There Ain't No Black in the Union Jack*, Hutchinson.

Goldson, E., Lavallette, M. and McKechnie, J. (2000) *Children, Welfare and the State*, Sage.

Gordon, L. (1989) *Heroes of Their Own Lives. The Politics and History of Family Violence, Boston, 1880–1960*, Virago.

Gorz, A. (1982) *Farewell to the Working Class? An Essay in Post-industrial Socialism*, Pluto.

Gramsci, A. (1978) *Selections from Political Writings 1921–1926*, Lawrence and Wishart.

—— (1986) *Selections From the Prison Notebooks*, Lawrence and Wishart.

Hall, S. (1988) 'The toad in the garden – Thatcherism among the Tories', in Nelson, C. and Grossberg, R. (eds) *Marxism and the Interpretation of Culture*, Macmillan.

Hall, S., Critcher, C., Jefferson, T., Clarke, J. and Roberts, B. (1978) *Policing the Crisis: Mugging, the State and Law and Order*, Macmillan.

Hallett, C. (1989) 'Child abuse inquiries and public policy', in Stevenson, O. (ed.) *Child Abuse, Public Policy and Professional Practice*, Harvester Wheatsheaf.

Hanmer, J. and Stathem, D. (1988) *Women and Social Work – Towards a Women Centred Practice*, Macmillan.

Hendrick, H. (2003) *Children, Childhood and English Society*, Cambridge University Press.

Heywood, J. S. (1978) *Children in Care – The Development of Services for the Deprived Child*, Routledge and Kegan Paul.

Hill, M. and Tisdall, K. (1998) *Children and Society*, Prentice Hall.

HMSO (1923) *First Report of the Home Office Children's Branch*, HMSO.

—— (1925a) *Report of the Departmental Committee on Sexual Offences Against Young Persons*, Cmnd 2831, HMSO.

—— (1925b) *Third Report of the Home Office Children's Branch*, HMSO.

—— (1927) *Report of the Departmental Committee on the Treatment of Young Offenders*, Cmnd 2831, HMSO.

HMSO (1933) *Children and Young Persons Act*, HMSO.
—— (1938) *Fifth Report of the Home Office Children's Branch*, HMSO.
—— (1965) *The Child, the Family and the Young Offender*, Cmnd 2742, HMSO.
—— (1968) *Children in Trouble*, Cmnd 3601.
—— (1987a) *Report of the Inquiry into Child Abuse in Cleveland 1987*, Cmnd 412, HMSO.
—— (1987b) *The Law on Child Care and Family Services*, Cmnd 62, HMSO, Home Office.
Horkheimer, M. and Adorno, T. (1972) *Dialectics of Enlightenment*, Herder and Herder.
Houghton Committee (1972) *Report of the Departmental Committee on the Adoption of Children*, Cmnd 5107, HMSO.
Ingleby Committee (1960) *Report of the Committee on Children and Young Persons (The Ingleby Report)*, Cmnd 1191, HMSO.
Jameson, F. (1988) 'Cognitive mapping', in Nelson, C. and Grossberg, L. (eds) *Marxism and the Interpretation of Culture*, Macmillan.
Johnson, I. T. J. (1972) *Professions and Power*, Macmillan.
Jones, C. (1976) 'An analysis of the development of social work and social work education 1869–1977', unpublished doctoral thesis, University of Durham.
—— (1983) *State Social Work and the Working Class*, Macmillan.
Kerns, D. L. (1989) 'Cool science for a hot topic', in *Child Abuse and Neglect*, 13: 179–93.
Laming, Lord (2003) *The Victoria Climbié Inquiry: Report of an Inquiry by Lord Laming*, Cmnd 5730, The Stationery Office.
Langan, M. and Lee, P. (1989) 'Whatever happened to radical social work?', in Langan, M. and Lee, P. (eds) *Radical Social Work Today*, Unwin Hyman.
Larrain, J. (1979) *The Concept of Ideology*, Hutchinson University Library.
Larson, M. S. (1977) *The Rise of Professionalism*, University of California Press.
Leeding, A. E. (1976) *Child Care Manual for Social Workers*, 3rd edn, Butterworth.
Lenin, V. I. (1963) *What Is To Be Done?* Clarendon Press.
Leonard, P. (1975) 'Towards a paradigm for radical practice', in Bailey, M. and Brake, R. (eds) *Radical Social Work*, Arnold.
—— (1984) *Personality and Ideology – Towards a Materialist Understanding of the Individual*, Macmillan.
London Edinburgh Weekend Return Group (1980) *In and Against the State*, Pluto Press.
Macdonald, G. (2001) *Effective Interventions for Child Abuse and Neglect – An Evidence-Based Approach to Planning and Evaluating Interventions*, John Wiley and Sons Ltd.
Marx, K. (1890) *Capital – Volume 1*, Progress Publishers.
Meiksins Wood, E. (1986) *The Retreat from Class*, Verso.

Milliband, R. (1989) *Divided Societies – Class Struggle in Contemporary Capitalism*, Oxford University Press.

Mitchell, J. (1975) *Psychoanalysis and Feminism*, Penguin, Harmondsworth.

Moore, J. (1985) *The ABC of Child Abuse Work*, Gower.

Muncie, J. and Hughes, G. (2002) 'Modes of youth governance – political rationalities, criminalization and resistance', in Muncie, J., Hughes, G. and McLaughlin, E. (eds) *Youth Justice – Critical Readings*, Sage Publications.

Neale, B. (2004) 'Young children's citizenship', in Willow, C., Marchant, R., Kirby, P. and Neale, B. (eds) *Young Children's Citizenship – Ideas into Practice,* Joseph Rowntree Foundation.

Parton, N. (1985) *The Politics of Child Abuse*, Macmillan.

—— (1990) 'Taking child abuse seriously', in The Violence Against Children Study Group, *Taking Child Abuse Seriously*, Routledge.

—— (1991) *Governing the Family – Child Care, Child Protection and the State*, Macmillan.

—— (2004) 'From Maria Colwell to Victoria Climbié: reflections on public inquiries into child abuse a generation apart', *Child Abuse Review*, 13: 80–94.

Pinchbeck, I. and Hewitt, M. (1973) *Children in English Society, Volume II: The Eighteenth Century to the Children Act 1948*, Routledge and Kegan Paul.

Pitts, J. (1988) *The Politics of Juvenile Crime*, Sage.

Poster, M. (1984) *Foucault, Marxism and History (Mode of Production versus the Mode of Information)*, Polity Press.

Rabinow, P. (ed.) (1986) *The Foucault Reader*, Peregrine Books.

Riley, D. (1983) *War in the Nursery – Theories of the Child and the Mother*, Virago.

Roderick, R. (1986) *Habermas and the Foundations of Critical Theory*, Macmillan.

Rojek, C., Peacock, G. and Collins, S. (eds) (1988) *Social Work and Received Ideas*, Routledge.

—— (1989) *The Haunt of Misery – Critical Essays in Social Work and Helping*, Routledge.

Schutz, A. (1966) 'Some structures of the life world', in Luckman, T. (ed.) (1978) *Phenomenology and Sociology*, Penguin Books.

Simpkin, M. (1983) *Trapped Within Welfare – Surviving Social Work*, Macmillan.

Sinclair, I. and Corden, J. (2005) *A Management Solution to Keeping Children Safe – Can Agencies on their Own Achieve What Lord Laming Wants?* Joseph Rowntree Foundation.

Sinclair, R. and Bullock, R. (2002) *Learning from Past Experience – A Review of Serious Case Reviews*, Department of Health.

Sivanandan, A. (1990) *Communities of Resistance – Writings on Black Struggles for Socialism*, Verso.

Smart, B. (1983) *Foucault, Marxism and Critique*, Routledge and Kegan Paul.

Smith, F. (1991) *Personal Guide to the Children Act 1989*, Children Act Enterprises.

—— (2005) *The Children Act 2004*, Children Act Enterprises.

Smith, S. (1989) *The Politics of 'Race' and Residence*, Polity Press and Basil Blackwell.

Smolen, K. (1982) *Auschwitz 1940–1945, Guide Book to Museum*, Krajowa Agencja Wydawnicza.

Solomos, J. (1989) *Race and Racism in Contemporary Britain*, Macmillan.

Stevenson, O. (ed.) (1989) *Child Abuse Public Policy and Professional Practice*, Harvester Wheatsheaf.

Terry, J. (1979) *A Guide to the Children Act 1975*, Sweet and Maxwell.

Therborn, G. (1980) *The Power of Ideology and the Ideology of Power*, Verso Editions and NLB.

United Nations Committee of the Rights of the Child (2002) – *Consideration of the Reports Submitted by States Parties Under Article 44 of the Convention – Concluding Observations: United Kingdom of Great Britain and Northern Ireland (CRC/15/Add.188)*.

United Nations Office of the High Commissioner for Human Rights (1989) *Convention on the Rights of the Child – Adopted an Opened for Signature, Ratification and Accession by General Assembly Resolution 44/25 of 20 November 1989 – Entry into Force 2 September 1990*.

Urwick, E. J. (1904) 'A school of sociology', in Loch, C. S. (ed.) *Methods of Social Advance*, Macmillan.

Vernon, S. (1990) *Social Work and the Law*, Butterworth.

Weber, M. (1948) in Wright Mills C. and Gerth, H. (eds) *Essays in Sociology*, Routledge and Kegan Paul.

Williams, F. (2000) 'Principles of recognition and respect in welfare', in Lewis, G., Gewirtz, S. and Clarke, J. (eds) *Rethinking Social Policy*, Sage.

Winnicott, C. (1984) *Child Care and Social Work – A Collection of Papers Written Between 1954 and 1963*, Bookstall Publications.

Winnicott, D. (1971) *Playing and Reality*, Penguin Books.

Wood, E. M. (1986) *The Retreat from Class: A New 'True' Socialism*, Verso.

Wyatt, G. and Higgs, M. (1991) 'The medical diagnosis of child sexual abuse: The paediatrician's dilemma', in Richardson, S. and Bacon, H. (eds) *Child Sexual Abuse: Whose Problem*, Venture Press.

Younghusband, E. (1947) *Report on the education and training of social workers*, Constable.

Index

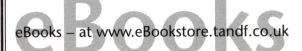